In Pursuit of Memory

In Pursuit of Memory

The Fight Against Alzheimer's

JOSEPH JEBELLI

JOHN MURRAY

First published in Great Britain in 2017 by John Murray (Publishers)
An Hachette UK Company

1

© Joseph Jebelli 2017

Illustrations by Matteo Farinella

A CIP catalogue record for this title is available from the British Library

Hardback ISBN 978-1-47363-573-9
Trade paperback ISBN 978-1-47363-574-6
Ebook ISBN 978-1-47363-575-3

Typeset in Bembo by Palimpsest Book Production Limited,
Falkirk, Stirlingshire

Printed and bound by Clays Ltd, St Ives plc

John Murray policy is to use papers that are natural, renewable and
recyclable products and made from wood grown in sustainable forests.
The logging and manufacturing processes are expected to conform to the
environmental regulations of the country of origin.

John Murray (Publishers)
Carmelite House
50 Victoria Embankment
London EC4Y ODZ

www.johnmurray.co.uk

For my grandfather

Contents

PART IV: Experimentation

PART V: Discovery

Preface: 'A Peculiar Disease'

Science is public, not private, knowledge.
Robert King Merton, *Science, Technology and
Society in Seventeenth-Century England*, 1988

W HEN I WAS twelve years old, my grandfather began to act strangely. I had known Abbas Jebelli as a self-effacing man, whose strong sense of family frequently carried him from volatile Iran to our quiet street in Bristol, England. He used to arrive with suitcases filled with pistachio nuts and Persian sweets, smiling until the corners of his eyes wrinkled as he handed us our gifts.

It started with inexplicable walks. When he was visiting, he'd leave the dinner table and then we would find him, half an hour later, aimlessly wandering the neighbourhood. '*Please* stop doing that,' my father would say. '*Bebakhshid*,' ('forgive me') was all Abbas ever replied in his native Farsi. His bright smiles were gradually replaced by a fearful, withdrawn expression, as if he'd lost something irreplaceable. Before long, he didn't recognise his own family.

Something indefinably peculiar had happened to him.

As far as I knew, though, Abbas was just getting old. For decades, human lifespan had been rising. In the 1940s you'd be lucky to make it to age fifty, my father had explained, but we're now living in the 1990s and Granddad was a leathery seventy-four-year-old whose mind, like his sight and nearly everything else, was slowly wearing out.

But that explanation never felt right. My young mind had no notion yet of the endless intricacies of the human brain, of the 85 billion cells that knit fragments of the past together into a ghostly tapestry that we call memory. Perhaps it was the sheer indiscriminateness of this bizarre affliction. Why, if this was 'normal', was my grandmother not going through the same thing? Why was the Queen still able to make such eloquent speeches on television when Abbas couldn't even draw a clock face? Why, for that matter, wasn't *everyone* who reached old age experiencing this?

Seventeen years later, I am standing in a small, dimly lit room in the Institute of Neurology at University College London. Glass beakers, pipettes, shelves filled with chemicals and reagents, and a large grey centrifuge surround me. The air is filled with the stinging scent of ethanol, and there's a quiet hum as curtains of sterile air separate me from the nearby workstations. I stare into a small light microscope, focusing the image until the contours of numerous circular entities come into view. These are brain cells, taken from a rat, which I'm hoping will make some sense of what happened to my grandfather and millions of others just like him – all stricken by one of the most terrifying illnesses of modern times: Alzheimer's disease.

The cells I'm looking at were already sick when I plated them two weeks ago; they've come from animals engineered to have the disease inscribed in their DNA. As expected, the now infamous plaques – dark patches that appear in the brains of Alzheimer's patients, proposed to be the disease's root cause twenty-five years ago – have started to form between them. But hidden among this neurological nightmare are the brain's immune cells, microglia. And if the immune stimulant I've given them works, they could unleash a potent chemical attack on the plaques, physically engulfing and degrading them in a cellular defence mechanism called phagocytosis. Whether they will, though, still remains a question.

This theory is one of many that scientists are now testing, for Alzheimer's is already a disease of global significance. It affects 47 million people worldwide and more than 800,000 in the UK alone.[1] As the world's population ages, Alzheimer's is expected to affect 135 million people by 2050, overtaking cancer to become the second leading cause of death after heart disease.[2] We've now reached a point at which almost everyone knows someone – whether a family member or a friend – who has been affected.

In recent years, cases from the echelons of high society have reached our ears as well. Rita Hayworth, Peter Falk, Charlton Heston, Rosa Parks, Margaret Thatcher – all eventually developed Alzheimer's. When President Ronald Reagan was diagnosed, in November 1995, he published a handwritten letter to the American public: 'At the moment I feel just fine. I intend to live the remainder of the years God gives me on this earth doing the things I have always done . . . Unfortunately, as Alzheimer's disease progresses, the family often bears a heavy burden. I only wish there was some way I could spare Nancy from this painful experience.'[3]

As anyone who has known a patient understands, Alzheimer's is a merciless disease. It strips the mind of decades of stored memories that have been sculpted and embedded deep within our brains. Slowly and steadily, it erodes an individual's autobiography, the very narrative that defines who we are. In his book *The Emperor of All Maladies*, Siddhartha Mukherjee describes cancer as 'a distorted version of our normal selves', 'an individual – an enigmatic, if somewhat deranged, image in a mirror'.[4] Perhaps, using this analogy, Alzheimer's is the absence of a reflection altogether – a shadowy abyss that disengages a person from the world.

When I set out to study Alzheimer's, it was for personal reasons. I never expected to cure the malady myself, but I did want to understand what happened to my grandfather after having to watch his memory disappear in this way. I learned quickly that the science behind the disease is still shrouded in mystery. Professor Alois Alzheimer, the eponymous German psychiatrist who first described it in 1906, called it 'a peculiar disease'. He was referring mainly to its underlying pathology. Through the microscope Alzheimer had observed numerous plaques and tangles of an unknown substance.

But he didn't know whether they were the disease's root cause or just an after-effect. This question has remained unanswered, and we still know very little about what causes brain cell death on such a massive scale.

Here is what we do know. A person with Alzheimer's is not 'just getting old'. Their brain is under attack. A host of killer proteins has been unleashed – insidious black stains known as plaques and tangles. After gestating in the brain for years, perhaps decades, they will spread and hollow it out. In the hippocampus, a brain region crucial for memory, the plaques start by destroying the brain's ability to create new memories by disrupting the electrical signals between neurons. As they grow in number, the plaques eventually trigger the rise of tangles – deformed proteins that completely unravel the neurons' internal transport mechanism. The ensuing neurotoxic storm then causes the brain's immune system to activate. But the damage is irreparable, and even our brain's best efforts to remedy the affliction are insufficient. One by one, like a chain of dominoes, neurons continue to fall. In only a few years after symptom onset, neurons in the frontal lobe and cerebral cortex will start to perish, disrupting mood, spatial awareness, face-recognition and long-term memory. Six to eight years is usually how long it takes. The result is a brain the weight of an orange, having shrunk at three times the rate of normal ageing.

But there is hope. Today, advances in genetics and cell biology are changing the conceptual landscape of Alzheimer's disease. Research has become highly collaborative: last year, for instance, more than 200 researchers from across Europe and the US worked together on a genetic study using 70,000 patients.[5] The effort uncovered eleven new genes linked to Alzheimer's disease, and armies of scientists continue to mobilise around the world in a concerted effort to unmask and disarm it. This book is, in part, a look at the fascinating and utterly important work they are doing.

But this wasn't enough for me. As time went on – as I moved through the ranks of postgraduate training, earning a doctorate in neuroscience and then becoming a postdoctorate researcher conducting independent research on neurodegeneration and mentoring my own students – I became convinced that studying Alzheimer's would require something more than what I could discover in the laboratory. A paradox of biological research is that its practitioners invariably succumb to a strange form of tunnel vision: the more we delve into a problem, the more sheltered we are from its wider reach. I wanted to meet other people like my grandfather and his family, dealing with Alzheimer's here and now, to tell the human story of this disease along with the scientific one.

Because more than anything, Alzheimer's is a disease that affects families. Its symptoms engulf those around it, causing emotional turmoil for family members who can do nothing but watch while their loved ones – hearts still pumping, breath still flowing, eyes still open – slowly slip away for ever. I wondered how others were coping with this. Did their stories bear any resemblance to what my own family went through? To find answers, I reached out to patients and families affected by the illness, including people with early-onset Alzheimer's who, after inheriting it from their parents, have had to make unimaginable decisions and sacrifices throughout their lives.

One of the first patients I met was eighty-four-year-old Arnold Levi. Arnold represents a typical case of Alzheimer's, and I listened as he and his carer, Danie, described the frighteningly tangible implications of this attack on Arnold's brain. It happened slowly at first. He'd forget the same kind of things many elderly people do: names, dates, paying the bills, stocking the fridge. Small things. Ordinary things. No one thought much of it, least of all Arnold. But over the course of a few years people *did* start to think about it. His friends noticed an intense and unshakable decline in his behaviour. He needed help getting dressed. He left taps running, the burner on the stove on, the front door unlocked. And of course, he wasn't trusted to drive any more.

And this was just the start. Over the next few years Arnold will become increasingly confused and agitated. His soaring level of forgetfulness and plummeting cognitive faculties will deeply frustrate him. Familiar people will seem like complete strangers. He may even frantically push them out the house, petrified by the 'intruder'.

Eventually, Arnold will no longer be able to speak, eat, drink or swallow. The most a loved one can hope for from the bedbound sufferer is the slightest quiver of comprehension from a tender touch or a cherished voice. Utterly robbed of his final years of life, Arnold will likely die of malnutrition or pneumonia, his mind now powerless to uphold the most primal rules of survival.

This is the horrifying reality of Alzheimer's. Scientists talk about Alzheimer's like detectives solving a crime – evidence versus speculation, deduction versus assumption, truth versus deception. We gather every clue we can before the brain cells we are studying vanish into thin air. At scientific meetings we ask questions about caveats and statistical significance. But Alzheimer's isn't like this for families. For us, it's something terrifying and abstract: an invisible thief, a long goodbye we now know is not just old age, but of which many people know little else. Meeting these families, I realised that they wanted answers from me as badly as I did from them.

One thing was clear: if they were going to enlighten me, I'd make sure I returned the favour. Intensely, I started reading everything I could about the disease. My desk filled with stacks of research articles and academic papers. My inbox flooded with emails about the news and contents of the most august scientific journals. I contacted all my scientific colleagues to learn how the field was changing, and to keep pace with the lightning speed of research. I travelled across the globe, visiting different laboratories, interviewing scientists and talking to patients and their families. I've had memory testing myself. I put all my powers of critical thinking from ten years of scientific training to the test. I was, in short, obsessed.

This is a book about the past, present and future of Alzheimer's. I started my investigation from the very beginning, from the first recorded case more than 100 years ago, right up to the cutting-edge research being done today. It is a story as good as any detective novel. It took me to nineteenth-century Germany and post-war England; to the jungles of Papua New Guinea and the technological proving grounds of Japan; to America, India, China, Iceland, Sweden and Colombia; and to the cloud-capped spires of the most elite academic institutions. Its heroes are expert scientists from around the world – many of whom I have had the privilege of working with – and the incredibly brave patients and families who have changed the way scientists think about Alzheimer's, unveiling a pandemic that took us centuries to track down, and, above all, reminding everyone never to take memory – our most prized possession, the faculty Jane Austen called 'more wonderful' than the rest – for granted.

Abbas didn't live long with his illness. In Iran, like a candle burning itself out, his mind faded and vanished within seven years. It had reached an unknown destination, a place every patient I spoke to was heading and somewhere one in three people born in 2015 is bound for as well.[6] I think about that nearly every day. It's what has driven me forward.

Author's Note

THE STORIES IN this book are real stories. Some patients have already received public attention for their illness and so were happy for me to use their real names. However, for reasons of anonymity, and because Alzheimer's disease remains stigmatised in some parts of the world, other patients requested privacy. In these instances I have changed their names and identifying details. I ask the reader to respect their right to confidentiality.

PART I

Origins

I

The Psychiatrist with a Microscope

Idle old man,
That still would manage those authorities
That he hath given away! – Now, by my life,
Old fools are babes again . . .

William Shakespeare, *King Lear*

HEN HE FINISHED his talk, Alois turned to the audience. There were nearly 100 guests in attendance, which usually assured a lively discussion. Alois – frank and commanding with a stout face, coiffed moustache, piercing gaze and immense stature – waited confidently. But no one spoke. Had they not understood him? Sensing an uncomfortable silence, the chairman intervened: 'So there, respected colleague Alzheimer, I thank you for your remarks, clearly there is no desire for discussion.'

It was 3 November 1906. Dr Alois Alzheimer, a psychiatrist in Munich, was at the South-West German Psychiatrists' meeting in Tübingen to describe a fifty-six-year-old woman with a peculiar and unexplained mental disorder. Her name was Auguste Deter.

Auguste had been brought to Alzheimer four years earlier by her husband Karl, a railroad worker who had spent the last eight months watching his wife's behaviour deteriorate. The couple had been married for twenty-eight years, had one daughter, and were living a normal, healthy and happy life together.

But things changed when Auguste became inexplicably paranoid about the relationship between Karl and their female neighbour.

3

More disturbing still was Auguste's severe decline in memory. She was the epitome of a good German housewife, and so it struck Karl as highly unusual when she started neglecting her housework and making mistakes in the kitchen. Over the next few months Auguste wandered aimlessly round their apartment, hiding family possessions and speaking ominously of death. Her delusions resulted in panic when she started to believe that a carriage driver was trying to break into the apartment.

Karl was bewildered. At the time illnesses like this were extremely uncommon in someone of Auguste's age, and overall rare in the population because living much beyond your sixties in 1901 was a rarity in itself. At a loss, Karl took his wife to one of the most highly regarded psychiatric clinics in the world: the Asylum for the Insane and Epileptic in Frankfurt, which had a nickname indicative of the attitudes towards mental illness at the time: 'The Castle of the Insane'.

Auguste's illness is the first reported case of what we now know as Alzheimer's disease, the most common cause of dementia. Dementia is an umbrella term encompassing a constellation of brain disorders – such as vascular dementia, Lewy body dementia and fronto-temporal dementia – all of which involve a gradual loss in several aspects of cognition including memory, language, attention, orientation and problem solving. It often manifests as personality changes, depression, paranoia, agitation, delusions and even hallucinations.

The sheer breadth of faculties under assault fosters much confusion when faced with an Alzheimer's victim. This was certainly true when it came to my grandfather. His four children, including my father, never truly accepted his diagnosis. They maintained that Abbas could be a curmudgeonly and somewhat eccentric character. They only recognised the term Alzheimer's as something abstract – a hazy miscellany of a crumbling mind. Our family certainly had little concept of a cause of dementia, let alone the existence of dementia subtypes. We know now that to say someone has dementia is like saying they have cancer without identifying which type of cancer. And so, just as melanoma is a type of cancer, Alzheimer's is a type of dementia.

We now know that Alzheimer's is distinguished from other dementias by its unique effect on parts of the brain that control thought and memory, as well as its characteristic pattern of structural and chemical changes that can be seen with brain imaging and post-mortem examinations – appearing as catastrophic nerve cell death, and plaques and tangles of toxic proteins scattered throughout the brain. Plaques, in pure biological terms, are sticky proteins that clump together in the spaces between nerve cells. Tangles are also clumps of sticky proteins, but they form inside nerve cells and are more threadlike in appearance. Both are thought to be a kind of molecular 'garbage' that distorts healthy brain function and ultimately leads to Alzheimer's. In truth, however, we're still not entirely sure what they are, why they form, or how they cause the disease. This urgently needs to change. According to the World Health Organization (WHO), Alzheimer's is now estimated to account for 70 per cent of all cases of dementia.[1]

But it took a long time to get this far.

For centuries, mental illness was thought to be the work of spirits and gods. In the book of Deuteronomy, the ancient Hebrews interpreted disordered thoughts as a curse from God for all who disobey Him: 'The Lord will strike you with madness and blindness and confusion of mind.'[2] Dementia was so poorly understood it was regarded along similar lines: those who had it were mad or just foolish. It was a time when unfounded beliefs held sway, and people tried to treat such illnesses by 'trepanation', drilling holes into the skull to release evil spirits. Greek and Roman philosophers sought to bring about a change through observation and scientific rationalism.

One of the earliest accounts of what we could call dementia was by the sixth-century BC mathematician Pythagoras, who described it as an inevitable outcome of old age; a period, in his words, where 'the scene of mortal existence closes, after a great length of life, to which, very fortunately, few of the human species survive. The system returns to the imbecility of the first epoch of infancy.'[3] The word 'imbecility' came from the Latin *imbecillus*, meaning 'weak-minded'. According to Pythagoras, human life followed the seasons – old age is winter, and so its changes, however severe or unpleasant, were natural. But others thought there was more to it.

Cicero, the Roman philosopher, was among the most vital advocates in this regard. He thought dementia affected 'only those who are weak in spirit and will'.[4] A misguided theory of course, but it was the first whisper of the notion that dementia is not an inevitable product of old age. He took things further by suggesting that exercise might even prevent such decline, which was highly progressive given what I discuss later in this book. Building on his work, the Greek physician Aelius Galenus, better known as Galen, continued to buck conventional wisdom by describing patients suffering from what he called *morosis* (mental slowness), elderly people whose 'knowledge of letters and arts are totally obliterated. Indeed, they can't even remember their own names.'[5] Galen shattered the ancient, irrational views his predecessors had created, recasting dementia as a medical problem worthy of deeper investigation.

However, the period that followed was almost disastrous. The Middle Ages saw a return to supernatural explanations for disease – dementia was a test of faith, a devil to be exorcised, a 'conse-quence of the original sin',[6] and many sufferers were branded as witches. Even so, Christian-Judaeo beliefs also inspired a great deal of humanitarian thinking in the more enlightened. Brain diseases were looked upon with compassion and the care of the mentally ill became a religious obligation. Rational therapies, such as diets, baths and herbal medicines, came into practice: salad greens, barley water and milk, for example, were encouraged to replace red meat and wine; others endorsed a blend of aloes, black hellebore and colocynth.[7]

When the Enlightenment began, a string of discoveries in physics, chemistry and medicine – by Isaac Newton, Joseph Priestley, John

Dalton, Luigi Galvani, Alessandro Volta and Edward Jenner – pointed towards the possibility of physical explanations for mental phenomena. The French philosopher René Descartes thought that experiences make tiny pores in the brain like needles making a pattern of holes in a linen cloth.[8] David Hartley, the eighteenth-century English physician, claimed that nerve vibrations create sensations and memory, and that violent vibrations are the cause of mental illness.[9] These ideas were vague and incomplete, but they were free of mysticism and the supernatural.

A tipping point arrived when the French psychiatrist Philippe Pinel became the first to separate discrete types of mental disorders from the broad-brush label of insanity; it was not good enough, he said, to call these patients 'mad'. At the Bicêtre Hospital in Paris, Pinel called for compassion and non-violence when caring for the mentally ill. He spent hours talking to his patients and insisted that they be unshackled from their iron chains. Driven to study mental illness after the suicide of a close friend, Pinel used the term 'dementia' (*démence*, 'out of one's mind') in 1797, ushering in the modern age of psychiatry.[10] In 1838 his most talented student, Jean-Étienne Esquirol, fiercely denounced any remaining stigma: 'A demented man has lost the goods he used to enjoy; he is a wealthy person turned poor. An idiot, by contrast, has always been unfortunate and poor.'[11]

Twenty-six years later, on 14 June 1864, Alois Alzheimer was born.

Alzheimer grew up in the small Bavarian town of Marktbreit, a place of fairy-tale houses and cobblestone streets, Roman castles and Catholic jurisprudence. His father, Eduard Alzheimer, was a lawyer who had lost his first wife to puerperal fever. After a year of grieving Eduard married her sister, Theresia, and the couple had six children together. Alois was the eldest.

In 1883, aged nineteen, he was the first in his family to apply to medical school and obtained a place at the University of Berlin, where the world's brightest medical minds were already making history. It had been there, in 1858, that the humble-looking poly-math Rudolf Virchow made great leaps in our understanding of basic biology. Virchow argued that cells, the basic structural unit of all organisms, were the roots of all disease. 'The body,' he wrote, 'is a cell state in which every cell is a citizen. Disease is merely the conflict of the citizens of the state brought about by the action of external forces.'[12]

After five years of study surrounded by these ideas, Dr Aloysius 'Alois' Alzheimer was licensed to practise medicine for the German Empire. His interest was in psychiatry, so he applied for an intern position at the Frankfurt Mental Asylum and was chosen for the job on the same day the application was received. When Alzheimer arrived at the asylum there was certainly no shortage of work to be done. The director, Emil Sioli, desperately needed help after the asylum's sole medical assistant retired and the only relief doctor on duty had accepted a job offer elsewhere. The twenty-four-year-old Alzheimer was faced with 254 patients and one exhausted mentor.

Though magnificent from the outside, the inside of the asylum was anything but. Like most things German at the time, it aimed to set the standard for ingenuity and so imposed the modern 'non-restraint' principle of treating patients, designed by the English psychiatrist John Conolly for a more humane treatment of the mentally ill. Straitjackets were forbidden. But as Alzheimer found out, this approach was not without its downsides: non-restraint also meant no forced feeding, bathing or cleaning. And with so many patients and so few staff, conditions soon spiralled out of control. As Alzheimer mused:

> Everywhere cursing, spitting patients sat around in the corners, repulsive in their manner, peculiar in their dress, and completely inaccessible to the doctor. The most unclean habits were quite common. Some patients appeared with pockets filled with all sorts of waste, others had masses of paper and writing materials hidden all over the place and in big packets under their arms. When one had to finally follow the rules of hygiene and do something to get rid of the filth, one could not proceed without resistance and loud cries.[13]

Alzheimer immediately began to make changes. He introduced long baths where particularly uncontrollable patients could wind down; large consultation rooms where the doctors could talk and develop a dialogue with the patients; and special rooms designated solely for the microscopic examination of brain tissue. In this setting Alzheimer dived head first into research. Inspired by his years at Berlin University, he spent hours at the microscope, analysing hundreds of patient samples. The hunt for the biological origin of brain disease had begun.

But Alzheimer needed the right tools, and that's exactly what his like-minded peer, Franz Nissl, provided. A twenty-nine-year-old physician from Munich, Nissl had been working on a technique he had discovered as a medical student half a decade earlier. Using a variety of chemical dyes with exotic names such as cresyl violet and toluidine blue, Nissl stained thin slices of brain tissue to see if they would show structures in the brain never before seen. The images he produced were striking. The detail of individual nerve cells – their size, shape, position and internal components – were suddenly visible to the human eye in bright colour. The 'Nissl stain' became a sensation, and scientists around the world used it to reveal a host of different brain structures. Alzheimer himself described it as 'quite superb'.

With his transformation of the asylum, championing of the microscope, and a number of great thinkers by his side, Alzheimer's career flourished. He gave lectures around the country where he talked about bizarre patient cases and showed beautiful images of his latest microscopic examinations using the Nissl stain. His peers called him 'the psychiatrist with a microscope'.

In 1894 an extremely wealthy woman called Cecilie Geisenheimer, the widow of a diamond dealer, was bold enough to ask Alzheimer to marry her. Alzheimer had met her in Algeria, where he was sent to treat her husband, Otto Geisenheimer. Otto and Cecilie had been travelling around North Africa on a scientific expedition when he fell ill with general paresis (a neuropsychiatric disorder caused by late-stage syphilis). The situation was grave, and so Alzheimer, whose reputation now preceded him, was asked to accompany the couple back to Germany. They made it as far as the south of France before Otto died in a hospital in St Raphael. In the years that followed Alzheimer watched over Otto's widow and the couple became close. Cecilie was a 'highly educated woman with great heartfelt kindness', one of their granddaughters later remarked.[14] The couple were married on 14 February 1895, and had three children together. Alzheimer's happiness, both professionally and personally, had reached its peak.

Six years later, aged forty-one, Cecilie died of suspected kidney disease. Alzheimer was devastated. Life had been going so well for him but now he was left with three young children to raise alone. His unmarried sister, Elisabeth, took on the role.

Nine months passed. On 26 November 1901 the grief-stricken Alzheimer was working diligently at the asylum. He'd been burying himself in work, seeing more patients and working later into the night than ever before. Little did he know that the patient who would make his name echo through history was now sitting in front of him eating cauliflower and pork for lunch.

The newly admitted Auguste Deter intrigued Alzheimer. One minute she would appear calm and lucid, the next frightened and confused, roaming the ward and grappling other patients' faces. Alzheimer interviewed her extensively, asking her to identify a series of objects: a pencil, a book, a bunch of keys. These small confusions are often the things that stick in the mind of those who first notice the onset of Alzheimer's in a loved one: car keys are found in the fridge, clothing in the kitchen cabinet, objects like kettles and mail can disappear and then turn up somewhere completely unexpected. When asked to write down her name, Auguste began with 'Mrs' but would then forget the rest – something Alzheimer had never seen before. He first called it 'amnestic writing disorder'.

Over the next few months Auguste became increasingly disorientated, forgetful and mentally unhinged. Hauntingly, she would often look Alzheimer in the eyes and repeat the words: 'I have, so to speak, lost myself.'

Alzheimer was fascinated. Auguste's condition fitted previous descriptions of dementia, of a confused state that still had no better explanation than normal ageing. But surely, at fifty-one she was still too young for that. He examined her every day, looking for subtle clues in behaviour that could shed light on the underlying disturbance. But Auguste's condition deteriorated to the point where Alzheimer could no longer gain any meaningful insight. In May 1902 his final entry in her medical record reads: 'Auguste D. remains hostile, screams, and lashes out as soon as one tries to examine her. She also screams spontaneously and then often for hours, so that she has to be held in bed. As far as food is concerned, she no longer keeps to prescribed meal-times. A boil has formed on her back.'[15]

Having done all he could with such an impenetrable disorder, Alzheimer moved on. There was little he could glean while Auguste was still alive. And he had been offered a position in the clinic of world-renowned psychiatrist Emil Kraepelin, in Munich. After fifteen years, Alois left the Frankfurt Castle of the Insane.

It was a wise decision. Though only six years Alzheimer's senior, Kraepelin had gained international fame with the publication of various psychiatry textbooks in which he declared his conviction that all mental disorders are biological in origin – a conclusion Alzheimer had already been moving towards.

This idea, however, met resistance. The theories of Sigmund Freud had already taken hold of both the public and scientific imagination in Germany, and in doing so gave rise to a scientific factionalism that would ultimately cost Alzheimer his audience in November 1906. Sigmund Freud's imaginative and beautifully crafted ideas on how the mind works and why it becomes disturbed were highly alluring. Childhood repression, the Oedipus complex, the id, ego and superego were just some of the ingenious concepts Freud espoused to explain the source of psychiatric diseases – which, he claimed, could be completely remedied using the subtle art of psychoanalysis. And in a time where so little hope of a cure for mental illnesses existed, it was no surprise that the Austrian physician's new outlook enraptured so many.

Back in Frankfurt, Sioli kept a close eye on Alzheimer's most important patient. But Auguste's castaway mind had now come to the end of its journey. On 6 June 1906 Alzheimer was informed of her death. He requested that Auguste's brain be sent to him for a post-mortem at his new laboratory in Munich.

The first thing Alzheimer noticed from the small, soft, slightly off-white ball of tissue – now sitting on his laboratory bench – was just how small it was. There was a large loss of brain tissue throughout the cerebral cortex – the top layer of the brain – and this seemed to be the result of a catastrophic extinction of nerve cells. Bordering these biological ruins were also what looked like scars made up of other cell types. When Alzheimer peered down the microscope, the most perplexing omen of all appeared.

Peppered throughout the brain were dark particles of an unknown substance. They appeared to have nestled themselves in the spaces between nerve cells. Some were much larger than the surrounding cells, others smaller. And unlike the shrivelled form of dying brain cells, these particles possessed a rugged, patchy texture that clearly marked them as separate entities. What these particles – or plaques, as they later came to be known – consisted of, and where they came from, was a mystery. Alzheimer called them *aufbaum productif* ('build-up products').

What they did reveal, or at least highly suggest in his opinion, was genuine biological evidence for a brain disorder that had so far been considered purely psychological. More determined than ever, Alzheimer continued to examine the samples, in which he uncovered another intriguing peculiarity. Swarming within the debris of dead nerve cells was a second dark substance. This one was less lumpy and more threadlike in appearance. It took on the shape of variegated tangles of material that stretched out within the carcass of the deceased cell. But whether this was the same enemy in a different uniform, or a different species of adversary altogether, was not clear.

When Alzheimer showed his findings to Kraepelin the pair knew they were on to something. Clinically, Auguste's illness seemed like a form of dementia, but the deeply bizarre and unique pattern of pathology suggested it was a distinct disease in its own right. Eager to share the discovery with the world, Alzheimer started preparing for the South-West German Psychiatrists' meeting, which was only a few months away.

Voices murmured and chairs creaked as the growing throng of intellectual heavyweights took their seats in the old university hall. If Alzheimer was anxious about the presentation, he didn't let it show. This was a good thing considering his audience, which included the legendary Hans Curschmann, who discovered the inherited muscle-wasting disease known today as myotonic dystrophy; Robert Gaupp, who contributed groundbreaking work on psychosis through his study of the German mass murderer Ernst Wagner; and Carl Jung, the most loyal of Sigmund Freud's apostles and soon to be famous successor to Freudian psychology. But none of these men were as great a cause for shattered nerves as the chairman himself: Alfred Hoche, a man of unsavoury eminence who believed the mentally ill should be murdered if they offered no benefit to society (his charming ideas later extended to include the 'racially inferior', giving the Nazis scientific justification for their atrocities). Still, Alzheimer was confident his findings would provoke interest, and with a deep breath, he began his talk titled: 'On a Peculiar Disease of the Cerebral Cortex'.

> From a clinical perspective my Auguste D. case already offered such a distinctive clinical picture that it could not be classified among any of the known illnesses . . .
>
> . . . her memory was most severely disturbed. If one showed her objects, she generally named them correctly, but immediately afterward she forgot everything again . . .
>
> . . . spread over the entire cortex, especially numerous in the upper layers, one finds millet seed-sized lesions, which are characterised by the deposit of a peculiar substance in the cerebral cortex . . .
>
> . . . Taken all in all we clearly have a distinct disease process before us.[16]

The silence that followed was disappointing, but not surprising. Neuroscience was still in its infancy, and scientists were busy grappling with Freud's concepts of psychoanalysis. In fact the rest of the meeting was largely devoted to Freudian psychology, which provoked intense discussion. And though the chairman usually comes to the rescue when a speaker is put through such an embarrassment, it's no surprise the eugenically minded Hoche kept quiet. The minutes of the meeting described Alzheimer's talk as 'inappropriate for a brief report' – hardly the reception it deserved.

The truth is that science has a bad reputation when it comes to accepting new ideas. As scientists, we like to think we are calm, objective, unbiased champions of the evidence. But if that evidence changes the paradigm, it often squanders the life's work of many proud people. This is just as true today as it was back in 1906.

Alzheimer died in 1915 of heart failure at the age of fifty-one. In the years following the Tübingen meeting he continued his investigations and identified four other cases similar to Auguste. In 1910 Kraepelin acknowledged Alzheimer's efforts in his latest psychiatry textbook, *Handbook of Psychiatry*, where the term 'Alzheimer's disease' was used for the very first time.

The importance of Alzheimer's work cannot be overstated. By linking the physical state of Auguste's brain to the bewildering facts of her behaviour, Alzheimer challenged his peers to think differently. Instead of being rooted in psychology, he made it clear that dementia may reflect deeper riddles of biology. And whatever Alzheimer's disease was, it was a riddle that cried out almost literally for a solution.

2

Understanding an Epidemic

The historian of science may be tempted to exclaim that when
paradigms change, the world itself changes with them.

Thomas Kuhn, *The Structure
of Scientific Revolutions*, 1962

IN THE DECADES that followed the eponymous Bavarian's first
public description of Alzheimer's, scientists, pathologists and
psychiatrists were at loggerheads over what he had actually
discovered. Alzheimer had certainly found a unique pattern of brain
pathology with those 'peculiar' plaques and tangles scattered among
the debris of dead nerve cells.

The trouble, however, was that these so-called 'hallmarks' of
Alzheimer's disease were also found in the brains of people with
nothing mentally wrong with them whatsoever, provided they lived
long enough. In fact, post-mortems revealed that a quarter of people
over the age of sixty developed plaques and tangles, despite being
mentally well when they died. But Auguste Deter was only fifty-six.
Was her brain undergoing some kind of accelerated ageing? If so,
Alzheimer's life's work was on shaky ground, for one could hardly
call brain ageing a 'disease'.

And therein lay the problem. Unlike cancer, or infectious
diseases such as tuberculosis and smallpox, dementia appeared
to have no obvious aberration to target therapeutically, no malignant tumour or foreign pathogen to work on. It seemed as
though brain cells simply withered away by their own volition.

For many, this made the puzzle unsolvable. Just as the true causes of diseases were hidden by mythology and superstition during medicine's infancy, Alzheimer's disease was cloaked under the smokescreen of ageing.

Frustrated by this new wave of uncertainty, in the mid-1920s supporters of Alzheimer set out to confront the issue once and for all. If Alzheimer's was really a disease, the first thing to do was pin down the symptoms. One of Alzheimer's supporters was Ernst Grünthal, a Polish psychiatrist trained by Kraepelin and later forced to flee Germany because of his Jewish ancestry, who in 1926 described what he considered to be the most indispensible features of the disease. These included gradual memory loss, disturbance of perception, carelessness in work and appearance, disorientation as to place and time, loss of words and slurred speech, dulling of comprehension, extreme irritability, uncleanliness and disordered movements.[1]

But with such a motley array of symptoms it's no surprise that Grünthal's work didn't stand up well. Patients often had different shades of these symptoms, and the absence of some altogether. Mindful of this, other psychiatrists suggested that Alzheimer's and dementia were one and the same, the only difference being that the former is more severe and strikes younger than the latter. Others thought there existed multiple subtypes of Alzheimer's disease depending on the patient's personality and environment. Vague and arbitrary age limits for the disease started to emerge. Fifty-five was seen as the upper limit for it to be Alzheimer's, and anything above this was dementia. In the 1940s this was raised to sixty-five and then seventy; the boundaries were so blurred no one could agree how to categorise it.

Freud's followers seized on the paradox, using it to reassert the insignificance of biological root causes and instead stress the centrality of Freudianism. Dementia must be caused by 'factors of a more personal nature', said David Rothschild, an American psychiatrist trained in psychoanalysis, in 1941.[2]

The resulting confusion severely knocked the confidence of the Alzheimer school of thought, and threatened to send dementia research back to the dark ages during a time when psychiatric hospitals in Europe and America saw a dramatic rise in the total number of patients admitted with the disease. 'Our institutions promise to become in time vast infirmaries with relatively small departments for younger patients with curable disorders,' warned Richard Hutchings in his 1939 address as president of the American Psychiatric Association.

With an impending public health crisis, it became imperative to refocus the world's attention on the problem. The time had come to parachute in a new breed of scientist.

What the hell would I want to do that for? Michael Kidd thought as he left the meeting. He had gone to discuss his latest research findings on the retina – its simple yet elegantly arranged layers of cells captivated him – and now his mentor wanted him to study brains using a complicated new tool called the electron microscope.

It was October 1961. Kidd, a physician completing neuroscience research at University College London, was stubbornly recalcitrant to career advice. Educated in Ashford, a small town in Kent, Kidd had joined the Royal Air Force as an operating room assistant before studying medicine and then taking a research job at the prestigious university. With his contract coming to an end, his only option now was to apply for the job at Maida Vale Hospital in north London, where they wanted to use the new technology to study a form of dementia called Alzheimer's disease, whatever that was – he would have to look it up before the interview.[3]

Robert Terry was not as reluctant. Ten years older than Kidd, he had already spent several years in Paris learning how to use the microscope while training to become a pathologist. He had served during the Second World War in the 82nd Airborne Division. His colleagues described him as a 'tough', 'serious', 'no-nonsense' figure.[4] Now, at the Albert Einstein College of Medicine in the Bronx, New York, he was eager to test the microscope on something original. Which is exactly how he saw Alzheimer's – as an untouched challenge, something that (as far as he was aware) no one else in the field was looking at.

Standing ten feet tall and weighing half a tonne, the electron microscope looks more like the periscope of a naval submarine than a typical microscope. It's so large it requires its own room in most laboratories. Before its invention in the 1930s, scientists depended on the light microscope, invented by the Dutch biologist Antonie van Leeuwenhoek (who used it to discover red blood cells). The light microscope gathers light from the visible spectrum using a system of lenses and can magnify objects up to 1,000 times. But the electron microscope, invented by the German physicists Ernst Ruska and Max Knoll, uses a beam of electrons and can magnify objects up to 2 million times – a 2,000-fold increase from what was previously possible. In 1937 the Hungarian physicist Ladislaus Marton began using it to take pictures of biological specimens, publishing the first EM images of bacteria. Shortly afterwards, others captured shots of fly wings, viruses and skin cells.

For Alzheimer's research it was revolutionary. If light microscopy made brain cells look like a collection of planets in the night sky, the electron microscope provided a satellite to map the continents, mountain ranges and sprawling cities on each celestial body. The technique was firmly established in European and American laboratories just in time for Kidd and Terry to examine the detailed landscape of a brain with Alzheimer's.

Working separately, they took samples of brain tissue from living Alzheimer's patients and used the device to zoom in on the plaques and tangles.[5] Neither knew what to expect. As they carefully focused the shower of electrons, a dark and ghostly silhouette began to creep into view. The once distant and abstruse Alzheimer plaque no longer looked like a scatter of small innocuous particles. Now it was an enormous mass of black interwoven threads, crisscrossing chaotically like a mesh of barbed wire. Whatever this was, it certainly looked capable of spreading destruction. Fragments of nerve cells lay strewn in its wake, while other cells appeared to have been pierced by shards of the dark threads themselves.

Scanning the wreckage further, the microscopists soon landed on the odd tangles of material that appeared to choke the cells from the inside. And almost immediately it was clear these were a different kind of adversary. They twisted and coiled around themselves in a strikingly ordered manner, forming curious helices much like the DNA double helix discovered by James Watson and Francis Crick only one decade earlier.

'If you want to understand function,' Crick famously said, 'study structure.' In that vein Kidd and Terry began contemplating the atomic architecture of the plaques and tangles, comparing it with what was already known about how organic molecules behave. Unknowingly, they had just formed a crucial allegiance with the blossoming field of biochemistry.

Both microscopists were in agreement that the components of the plaques closely resembled a substance called amyloid. Coined by Rudolf Virchow in 1854, amyloid derives from the Latin *amylum*, for 'starch', combined with the Greek suffix *-oid*, meaning 'like' – Virchow had mistakenly identified the substance as a type of sugar. By the time Kidd and Terry began investigating, it had been discovered that amyloids are in fact composed of proteins.

Proteins are the chemical workhorses of life. Thousands of different kinds exist inside every cell in the body. Some are small and simple, performing routine tasks such as maintaining cell structure; others are large and complex, with multiple roles in tasks such as cell mobility, communication and protection from cancer. Built from a string of amino acids folded into an elaborate three-dimensional shape, proteins are the 'actors' of the cell while genes simply provide the 'script', or instructions, to create them. In other words, it is our genes that conceive of life but our proteins that construct it. But occasionally a protein will malfunction, go off radar, and settle as deposits in and around bodily organs. By the 1960s researchers started to notice an intriguing prevalence of these amyloid deposits in many disorders, including diabetes, kidney disease and certain heart conditions. Alzheimer's, it seemed, now had to be added to the list.

What the microscopists could not agree upon, however, was the structure of the tangles. Kidd, convinced by their striking resemblance to DNA, called them 'paired helical filaments'. Terry, on the other hand, believed each tangle to be a tube-shaped twist of material, which he called a 'twisted neurotubule'. I, for my part, often think they could be both after seeing them in the lab. It sounds trivial, but getting the answer right was critical – it was this kind of scrutiny that helped scientists understand how viruses behave.

For the next thirteen years neither microscopist could figure out which interpretation was right. Then, in 1976, using a combination of the latest electron microscope and advancements in biochemistry, Terry discovered that Kidd was right: the tangles were indeed a strange double-helical filament similar in structure to DNA.

Knowing the shape of the tangles was important because it made it clear they were fundamentally different from the plaques, which were spherical and contained stacks of amyloid piled on top of one another like rungs on a ladder. This laid the foundation for further questions about the relation of plaques and tangles. Which came first? Did one cause the other? And are they both necessary to cause the disease?

All that had to be done now was to remove the veil of ageing. 'Meeting the demand that senility be taken seriously involved reframing it as a scientific rather than a social problem,' wrote science historian Jesse Ballenger. 'Research had to be about more than the process of ageing; it had to be about something real and immediate – a dread disease.'[6] In other words, it didn't matter that Alzheimer's was associated with ageing. It was a disease that had to be recognised and clearly defined. To do this, though, a correlation between Alzheimer's and brain pathology had to check out: the scientists would have to prove that Alzheimer's could be seen and measured in the brain.

This was no easy feat. The biology of brain ageing remains among the deepest mysteries in neuroscience. Healthy brains shrink and lighten by roughly 10 per cent between the ages of fifty and eighty. Some brain cells die naturally as part of this process, but most simply shrink and function more slowly – which is why elderly people can experience mild forgetfulness and occasionally have trouble with words and everyday tasks. But it's still not clear why plaques and tangles can also accumulate during normal ageing. The greatest conundrum for early researchers, therefore, was how to square the fact that some people developed plaques and tangles while remaining Alzheimer's-free.

In 1966 an English research group at Newcastle University, led by Hungarian-born Martin Roth, devised a study to do just that. Roth believed that the main reason early attempts to link the plaques and tangles to the physical manifestation of Alzheimer's had failed was because we'd been approaching the problem in the wrong way. Performing post-mortems on brains first and then retrospectively trying to piece together a clinical picture of the patient while they were still alive was, he said, erroneous. It was also unscientific: the clinical picture of Alzheimer's patients was based on hospital notes, written by people who, despite their best efforts, would inevitably paint different pictures of the same patient. A more objective method was needed, one that could accurately measure a suspected case of Alzheimer's during life, follow the brain to post-mortem, and only then look for any biological correlations.

He recruited the help of pathologist Bernard Tomlinson and psychiatrist Gary Blessed, both of whom, like Roth, thought that dementia was being ignored largely because the methods for defining it were unsophisticated. The trio began by devising a 'dementia score': a test for assessing a patient's cognitive ability. Every six months they asked a patient's close relative to score their loved one on a battery of questions involving everyday habits, domestic tasks, personality changes and memory. For instance, how able were they to cope with small sums of money? Or remember lists of items on a shopping list? Could they eat and get dressed unaided? Did they remember the date of the Second World War? Or who the current Prime Minister was? Crucially, the study included elderly patients who were deemed cognitively normal in order to find out which symptoms were linked to Alzheimer's and which were just old-age forgetfulness. Once the brains came to post-mortem, the researchers counted the plaques, comparing the severity of plaque burden with the dementia scores they had collected over the final years of a patient's life.

The results spoke for themselves: there was an irrefutable connection between dementia scores and plaque count. The higher the former – you guessed it – the greater the latter. In a landmark paper published in *Nature*, Roth, Tomlinson and Blessed declared that, 'Far from plaques being irrelevant for the pathology of old-age mental disorder, the density of plaque formation in the brain proves to be highly correlated with quantitative measures of intellectual and personality deterioration in aged subjects.'[7]

More importantly, they found that ageing alone was not enough to explain the number of plaques seen in Alzheimer's patients. With an air of modesty that now seems overly cautious, they ended their report by asserting that: 'The facts suggest that [plaques] and related processes may also deserve investigation with the aid of more precise techniques than those employed in this study.'

The twentieth-century philosopher of science Thomas Kuhn observed that great scientific discoveries seldom occur in a steady, stepwise fashion. Instead, he said, they happen in 'paradigm shifts', in which 'one conceptual world view is replaced by another'.[8] Kidd and Terry's probing microscopy work, combined with Roth, Tomlinson and Blessed's great unveiling of a disease, did that for dementia. By depicting plaques and tangles in sharp relief against the rest of the brain, and combining innovation with careful examination and good science, they brought about a radical rethink in how we should define and approach the problem. They made it clear that people with Alzheimer's were suffering from an affliction no less urgent than cancer or stroke. And if people with other diseases of old age deserved recognition and action, then so did people with Alzheimer's. They had elevated a pursuit long considered futile.

Soon others started to speak out, including the physician and scientist Robert Katzman who, inspired by his mother-in-law's battle with the disease, became a staunch and leading activist for

Alzheimer's research. In a historic editorial published in 1976 in the *Archives of Neurology*, titled 'The prevalence and malignancy of Alzheimer's disease', he argued that the time had come to stop thinking of Alzheimer's and dementia as separate disease entities.

'Neither the clinician, the neuropathologists, nor the electron microscopist can distinguish between the two disorders, except by the age of the patient,' Katzman wrote. 'We believe it is time to drop the arbitrary age distinction and adopt the single designation, Alzheimer's disease.'[9] In this context, he proposed that Alzheimer's was a biological affliction that occurred along an age continuum. Rare cases appeared in middle age to sixty, with a predictably increasing likelihood for every ten years thereafter.

Many scientists agreed, and this new acceptance highlighted Alzheimer's as 'a major killer' – the fourth leading cause of death in America alone – and something far more ominous than previously thought. With the world's population steadily ageing, Alzheimer's could now be seen for what it truly is: a global and inescapable epidemic.

3

A Medicine for Memory

All life is chemistry.

J. B. van Helmont, *Ortas Medicinae*, 1648

O N 5 NOVEMBER 1986, in a proclamation to raise awareness for Alzheimer's, President Ronald Reagan addressed the crowd: 'No cure or treatments yet exist . . . but through research we hope to overcome what we now know is a disease . . .'[1] For the scientists who had worked for so long to prove that Alzheimer's is not a normal part of ageing, this public recognition of the Alzheimer's epidemic was a landmark moment. Three years earlier, President Reagan had declared November as America's National Alzheimer's Disease Month. Reagan would himself later succumb to Alzheimer's.

On the same November day in 1986, the office of William Summers, a neuroscientist at the University of Southern California, Los Angeles, was flooded with telephone calls from the press. They had in their possession an advance copy of the *New England Journal of Medicine* article that Summers was about to publish, which, he claimed, demonstrated a treatment for Alzheimer's disease.

Recent attempts to understand the brain have mainly involved breaking it down into its constituent parts, examining those parts, and then fitting them into a larger theoretical framework – a philosophy known as reductionism. Though many now believe it's time to move on from this way of thinking because the brain is proving more complicated than the sum of its parts, reductionism has provided us with an enormous amount of knowledge, upon which much of the research into a cure for Alzheimer's has relied.

Broadly speaking, the brain is composed of two main cell types – neurons and glia. Neurons, the nerve cells of the brain, are electrical cells that send chemical messages to one another at specialised contact points called synapses. They are often compared to trees in a dense forest or wires in a telecommunications network. You could also think of them as the masters of social media: each neuron is like a person that has around 85 billion 'friends', and they are part of a 'network' of synaptic connections that is 100 trillion strong. This means that every second, billions of neurons are sending trillions of synaptic messages in the deepest recesses of your mind.

Glia (Greek for 'glue') are non-electrical cells that protect and support neurons. It was thought they did little else – hence the disparaging Greek translation. But there is now good evidence that glia command far more illustrious roles in the brain, and swathes of neuroscientists on the front lines of Alzheimer's research are busy deciphering those roles in a bid to exploit them therapeutically.

According to the British biologist Lewis Wolpert, the best way to appreciate a neuron's complexity is to imagine each is the size of a human. At this scale the whole brain would cover an area of ten kilometres, nearing the size of Manhattan – and ten kilometres into the sky. The population of Manhattan is around 1.6 million people, but this space would be occupied by billions of 'neuron-people' piled high on top of one another, each one talking to between 100 and 1,000 of its neighbours.[2] If you can imagine that, then you can get a sense of how sophisticated the neuron is.

A typical neuron is composed of a cell body, numerous fine projections called dendrites, and one long projection called the axon. Several 'internal organs', or organelles, exist inside the cell body – such as the nucleus, which houses the neuron's DNA, the mitochondria, which provide the neuron with energy, and the ribosomes, which act as microscopic protein factories. Closely spaced

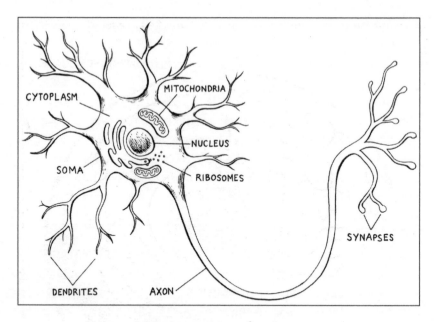

Major components of a neuron

along the length of the dendrites are the synapses, each one making contact with another neuron by almost touching the terminal of its axon. In this way neurons form a fixed but highly dynamic web of interactions.

Zooming out from this level, the brain is held together in distinct anatomical units, like pieces of glass in a stained-glass window. Each unit takes on the duty of controlling different functions.[3] The medulla oblongata, for instance, is located at the base of the brain-stem and performs the onerous task of regulating heart rate, blood pressure and breathing. The cerebellum, just above the brain stem, helps coordinate movement. The thalamus, buried deep within the centre of the brain, controls sleep and wakefulness. The cerebral cortex, that eye-catching folded outer layer of the brain, gives rise to the higher human faculties, such as language, emotion and consciousness. And the hippocampus (Greek for 'seahorse'), one of the very first regions to succumb to Alzheimer's, plays a pivotal role in converting short-term memory to long-term memory.

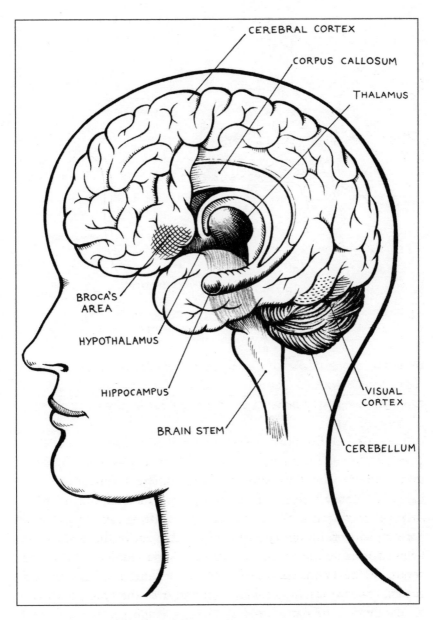

CEREBRAL CORTEX

CORPUS CALLOSUM

THALAMUS

BROCA'S
AREA

HYPOTHALAMUS

HIPPOCAMPUS

BRAIN STEM

VISUAL
CORTEX

CEREBELLUM

Examples of just a few brain regions

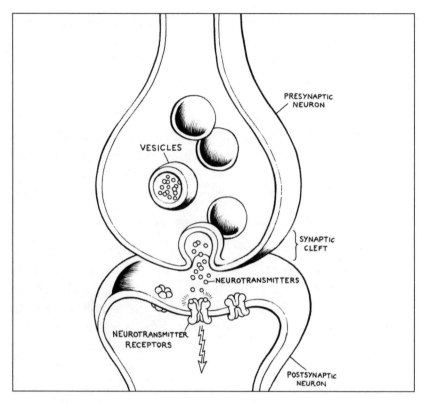

Neurotransmitter release at the synapse

The brain works by constantly transmitting chemical messages across synapses. When such a message is delivered, the neuron is said to have 'fired', resulting in countless different processes – from making sure you continue to breathe to ensuring your fingers do what you tell them to do. We call these messages neurotransmitters and most come in the form of chemical compounds. Glutamate, for instance, is a major neurotransmitter. Acetylcholine is another.

The signals these molecules convey form the roots of many aspects of normal brain function: emotion, learning, memory. While pinpointing a thought's origin in the brain is like deciding where a forest begins, thoughts are essentially generated by neurons triggering the release of neurotransmitters. It comes as no surprise, then, that scientists in the 1970s turned their heads when a striking loss of the neurotransmitter acetylcholine was seen in the brains of Alzheimer's patients.

It was 1978 and, almost simultaneously, three groundbreaking studies by separate teams of British biochemists were changing the face of Alzheimer's research: one led by Peter Davies at Edinburgh University;[4] the second by Elaine and Robert Perry at Newcastle University;[5] the third by David Bowen at the London Institute of Neurology.[6]

The 1970s were a fertile decade for dementia awareness. In America, Florence Mahoney, a prominent health activist, began lobbying politicians to create a new institute that specialised in age-related disorders to complement the already existing National Institute of Health (NIH). With her help, Congress convinced President Nixon to pass the Research on Aging Act of 1974, and a National Institute on Aging (NIA) was established. In the UK, health activist Peter Campbell founded the Mental Patients' Union (MPU), which campaigned against the then asylum-based psychiatric system that had been repeatedly exposed as a source of neglect and abuse for people with dementia,[7] and in 1979 a small group of patient relatives and prudent medical practitioners formed the Alzheimer's Disease Society (known today as the Alzheimer's Society). Across Europe, prestigious academic institutes – in Berlin, Paris, Rome and Stockholm – began to bring together scientists from diverse backgrounds and establish university departments with the sole purpose of unearthing the disorder's unknown origins.

In Britain, the biochemists had noticed a mysterious link between the effects of a childbirth anaesthetic and memory formation. From the turn of the century until the 1960s, a drug called scopolamine was used to spare mothers the pain of childbirth. Before that, chloroform had been the only option, but it was widely rebuked in the medical establishment as the source of life-threatening complications such as heart failure. Scopolamine, derived from the Asian flowering plant *Scopolia tangutica*, signified progress for its capacity to induce a 'Twilight Sleep': a state where the patient felt no pain while simultaneously remaining completely awake. More striking, though, was the intriguing observation that mothers often emerged from the treatment with no memory of their birthing experience whatsoever. No one could explain it. But what scientists did know was that scopolamine disrupted acetylcholine signalling in the nervous system.

Pinning down the neurochemistry of how memories are formed was, and remains, a Holy Grail for neuroscience. We still don't know how memory works. In the 1970s the Norwegian scientists Per Anderson and Terje Lømo had offered the most convincing theory to date. They argued that memories are made and lost by a respective strengthening and weakening of neuronal synapses. They called their model 'long-term potentiation' (LTP).[8] The phenomenon occurs, they said, after a synapse receives a high-frequency electrical stimulation. This causes a long-lasting increase in the strength of connections between neurons. Like almost everything in science, the truth (or in this case, the hypothesis) is almost too strange to comprehend, but Anderson and Lømo suggested that those connections – simply put – *are* our memories. They are nothing like how we perceive them to be – images and feelings passing through our minds. Memories are physically encoded.

So when a memory is born, say, from meeting someone for the first time, the information is first sent to the hippocampus to be encoded in a network of synapses. Some of this information will linger here as short-term memory, which lasts around thirty seconds, but if something about the meeting is important or has a strong emotional element, then the information is channelled to synapses in the cortex where it resides as long-term memory. If the science here sounds imprecise and unsatisfactory, that's because it is. We know that long-term memory can be divided broadly into declarative and procedural. Declarative memory refers to knowledge gathered over a lifetime, like the name of your dog, or how many children you have. Procedural memory involves remembering how to do certain things, like tying shoelaces, or driving a car. But in terms of memory's underlying neurophysiology, Anderson and Lømo's theory of LTP, combined with the observation that neurotransmitter signalling is somehow involved, was (and still is) the best description of memory in neuroscience.

With that, the British biochemists immediately asked the obvious question: could acetylcholine loss be the key to the decline in memory seen in Alzheimer's disease? It was a highly attractive theory. If proven true it could collapse the entire puzzle into a single piece: scientists would be able to develop a drug that simply replaces the acetylcholine. Indeed, Parkinson's research had triumphed this way in the 1960s, when a loss of the neurotransmitter dopamine was identified and scientists discovered a way to replace it using the drug Levodopa. Though not curative, the therapeutic gain for Parkinson's patients has been remarkable.

But in the case of Alzheimer's the answer was not so straightforward, and the success of the idea depended upon a number of questions. The first: was there a reduction in acetylcholine found in brain samples from deceased Alzheimer's patients? After an extensive search of post-mortem tissue the British groups were in unanimous agreement, and by 1978 all had published their findings. 'Yes', it appeared.

The next question: could artificially blocking acetylcholine in young healthy people trigger the same kind of memory loss seen in the elderly? As luck would have it this question had already been answered. In 1974 David Drachman and Janet Leavitt at Northwestern University, Chicago, took a group of young student volunteers, gave them a dose of 'Twilight Sleep' using scopolamine, and tested their ability to store and retrieve new memories.[9] Could they, for example, remember and repeat a random sequence of numbers after listening to them on a tape recorder? And how many nouns could they list that were categorised as animals, fruits and girls' names? They then gave the same tests to healthy volunteers aged between fifty-nine and eighty-nine who had not been given the drug. Astonishingly, while the untreated students far outperformed the elderly subjects in every test, the students under the influence of scopolamine performed just as poorly as their elderly counterparts. Here again, the answer was an affirmative.

The final question – and indeed the most crucial – was: does boosting acetylcholine release in the brains of living Alzheimer's patients improve their memory? The simplest way to test this was dietary. To make acetylcholine, neurons first need choline, a vitamin found circulating in the blood. The vitamin is provided in significant amounts from the food we eat – eggs, beef and fish, for instance, are plentiful in choline.

From 1978 to 1982 a number of European and American clinical trials tested the effect of dietary choline supplements on Alzheimer's patients.[10] They used doses up to fifty times the average human intake, gave it every day for months at a time, tested hundreds of patients of different ages, and implemented dozens of new methods for assessing memory and cognitive ability. The trials were the culmination of a collective effort of more than a dozen studies performed by a total of nearly 100 of the world's leading scientists. It hailed the first milestone in translating the findings of basic research into a real-world therapy for Alzheimer's. And it marked a new precedent in the history of humanity's response to the disease.

But it failed. The results of almost every study reported no effects on memory and no improvement on any tests of cognition. While a few groups declared some benefit, the data backing up such claims was inadequate. Whatever the reason, neurons had given up making acetylcholine, and giving them copious amounts of choline in the hope they would kick-start the mechanism back into action wasn't enough.

But all was not lost. 'Truth in science,' the Austrian zoologist Konrad Lorenz said, 'can be defined as the working hypothesis best suited to open the way to the next better one.' What if, some scientists asked, instead of trying to make new neurotransmitter from scratch, we simply kept the acetylcholine that was already present in the brain around for longer?

On the evening of 16 March 1988 huge clouds of yellow smoke began to rise into the air in the small city of Halabja, in the foot-hills of the Hawraman Mountains in Iraqi Kurdistan. Confused families rushed indoors and into basements; others ran into their cars and closed the windows. What they saw defied belief. In the streets among the smoke, crowds of people were uncontrollably vomiting, urinating and defecating, before violently convulsing and falling to the ground in seizures. The attack left an estimated 5,000 people, mostly civilians, dead, massacred by Saddam Hussein's forces in the final days of the Iran–Iraq war. The weapon of choice was a deadly chemical nerve gas known as sarin.

Sarin is twenty times more toxic than cyanide. It works by meddling with the neurotransmitter acetylcholine. Specifically, it binds to and paralyses another protein, called acetylcholinesterase, responsible for degrading acetylcholine. This causes a build-up of excess neurotransmitter, which wreaks havoc on the nervous system because acetylcholine signalling is also responsible for controlling muscle contraction. As a result the victim experiences a grotesque and undignified purge from every orifice before the muscles controlling their lungs fail, their chest tightens, and they eventually stop breathing altogether. Depending on the dose, death can occur within minutes.

The grim and lethal effect of sarin gas on humans was known long before the Iraqi massacre brought this horrifying reality to the world stage. As early as the 1950s its reputation as the deadliest nerve agent made the USSR and America begin stockpiling it for military purposes. So in 1981 when a neuroscientist named William Summers proposed using a drug that also works by binding and paralysing acetylcholinesterase to treat Alzheimer's patients, he trod carefully.

Summers was interested in a drug called tacrine (otherwise known as 1,2,3,4-tetrahydroacridin-9-amine). Synthesised by an

Australian chemist during the Second World War in a hunt to develop antiseptics for treating wounded infantry, tacrine was effectively shelved and forgotten to make way for penicillin. But animal tests using tacrine during the war effort revealed a curious property: it always counteracted the anaesthetic that scientists administered to an animal (usually a mouse) to put it to sleep. This intrigued another Australian, a psychiatrist named Sam Gershon, in the late 1950s. The arousing effect of tacrine appeared to stem from its ability to block acetylcholinesterase – making its behaviour similar to that of sarin gas but with a much less dangerous effect.

Raised on the wooded outskirts of a small town in central Missouri, Summers is a very different breed of scientist. His pragmatic yet unorthodox approach seems to have run in his family: both his father and grandfather were physicians and the young Summers, who was expected to follow in the family tradition, would often accompany them to the local hog-rendering plant to collect pig thyroids. The family would hang and dry the thyroids in their garden and then harvest the extract to treat patients with hypothyroidism – an effective method that was eventually replaced by synthetic means. Summers first became interested in Alzheimer's while training in psychiatry at Washington University in St Louis, when the idea of Alzheimer's as a form of dementia was beginning to take hold.

However, Summers remains unconvinced by the popular idea that plaques and tangles cause the disease. 'I think they just mark where the dead neurons are,' he told me, during a long conversation in the office of his private practice in Albuquerque, New Mexico. 'They might cause some neuronal death, but I think for the most part they're actually protective mechanisms against other things. There are probably more than fifty different targets and Alzheimer's is just the result of a final common pathway.' For Summers, acetylcholinesterase is the target – and tacrine the ideal weapon.

In February 1981 he administered the drug to twelve Alzheimer's patients intravenously.[11] The doses varied – after all, no one had any idea what amount would be effective, detrimental, or even fatal. But for all the suspense and trepidation the results were remarkably positive. Nine patients showed significant improvements in cognition only a few hours following treatment. And the side effects were mercifully limited to mild nausea and excessive sweating. 'It impressed me,' said Summers, 'that a toxin can, in the proper circumstances, become a medicine.'

Summers was eager to push his study further, but others in the hospital remained sceptical. As a full-time clinician at the University of Southern California the majority of Summers' working day was spent seeing patients, which left little time for research. Determined to pursue his research, Summers left the clinic and went into private practice: 'I thought what the hell, I would go earn money in the private sector, pay for my own research, and who gave a damn what they thought at the NIH!'

A straight-talking and resolute man by nature, Summers spent $90,000 out of his own pocket – $300,000 by today's standards – to develop a tacrine pill with the help of a few supporters at the University of California, Los Angeles (UCLA) and the Aldrich Chemical Company in Milwaukee. Mice and primates underwent testing, the US Food and Drug Administration (FDA) approved human trials, and by 1986 Summers published the results of seventeen patients given the drug orally in the *New England Journal of Medicine (NEJM)*.[12]

His findings were an instant sensation: the drug did appear to temporarily improve memory and cognition in Alzheimer's patients. It wasn't a cure, but for the millions watching loved ones slipping away, the beacon of light it offered was blinding. 'The genie was out of the bottle,' said Summers. 'There was a Saudi prince who had Alzheimer's and they were going to send a jet to LAX to pick me up and take me to Saudi Arabia to treat the prince. I had no idea what I was playing with to be honest.'

For all the excitement, though, there were many doubters. One troubling issue for the FDA and fellow neuroscientists was that Summers did the study out of his private psychiatric practice, under his own steam, out of sight of the academic establishment. This raised suspicion. Indeed, other researchers failed to replicate the result. Before long, Summers found himself embroiled in a year-long federal investigation.

'There's a rule of invention,' he told me, 'the lion's share of invention takes place in the wrong place, by the wrong people, at the wrong time, for the wrong reasons. I fit all of those. The discovery of the first treatment for Alzheimer's should certainly have come from the NIH, not from an individual in private practice in LA, and it should've come from big government grants, not from somebody who's self-funded on a shoestring.' The *NEJM* article, said the FDA, was overstated and misleading. According to them, there were gaping holes in the techniques and conclusions, reflecting an additional failure on the part of the *NEJM* reviewers.

Eventually, Summers was vindicated. A special committee of faculty at UCLA, charged with scrutinising his work with a fine-tooth comb, told the FDA that it checked out and on 10 September 1993 tacrine became the first FDA-approved treatment for Alzheimer's disease. As more patients started enrolling in the treatment it became clear that the effects – though positive – were modest. But it was enough to bolster hope in the idea that the disease would, and could, yield to treatment – something many in the broader scientific community never thought possible.

Today there are four internationally approved drugs for the treatment of Alzheimer's: Donepezil (Aricept™), Rivastigmine (Exelon™), Galantamine (Razadyne™), and Memantine (Namenda™). The first three work using the same scientific principle as tacrine. Patients who take them usually show a delay in the worsening of their symptoms for about six to twelve months – allowing them to cope better with simple daily tasks like dressing, shopping and personal hygiene. Whether you agree with Summers' somewhat renegade methods or not, he was a trailblazer for modern Alzheimer's research. His work created a desperately needed inroad of hope in a world with Alzheimer's disease rapidly on the rise. More importantly, his efforts signalled the first major assault on the disease that was based on a scientific, evidence-based hypothesis, giving other scientists the confidence to assert their own mechanistic theories. Would he do it again? 'Yeah, I'd do it in a heartbeat. Look at the people who have hope and are getting benefit. So it was worth every battle.'

We have entered a very different world from the one Summers and his predecessors entered. Their study of Alzheimer's taught us that memory is a material phenomenon, a subtle and exquisite product of healthy brain cells. They taught us that if memory resides anywhere, it resides in a network of durable connections and neurotransmitter systems between those brain cells. And if the rhythms of a damaged heart could be exposed and repaired, then so could memory. They had demonstrated that Alzheimer's could be abolished.

PART II
Research

FOR MY FATHER, the suspicion that Abbas was sick came during a phone call in the winter of 2003. My aunt Masoumeh had noticed that Abbas had forgotten where he lived. For weeks, she said, Abbas was either walking to the old family home in north Tehran, only to be turned away by its new residents, or he circled a nearby park, trying to piece together the details of his true address. When he did remember his way home, moreover, his wife Afsana was turning him away because he had been calling her 'Parry' – his first wife's name. My father encouraged her to take Abbas to the doctor. He knew how difficult the old man could be, but Abbas was behaving like a tourist in his own neighbourhood, and he had been 'newly' married for eighteen years.

Until then I still believed that Abbas's behaviour was normal and assumed that wouldn't change. But when my father put down the phone that day I knew that things were different. He booked a flight to Iran the next day.

Eight years later, I sat with my father at a dinner for Persian New Year in a hotel in central Bristol. A group of elderly Iranian expats were sitting on the next table, laughing, sipping tea, chatting about friends and family.

'You know, Dad,' I said as the waiter poured our drinks, 'I can't really remember a time when Granddad was like that.'

'You were young. He was a very sociable man before his Alzheimer's.'

'How did you find out he has Alzheimer's?'

'We took him for memory tests and a brain scan and the doctors said it was probably Alzheimer's.'

'*Probably* Alzheimer's,' I said, surprised by the flippancy of the description. 'What else did they say?'

'Not much, only that it was very difficult to know for sure.'

I wondered if that was still the case. At the time, I had just completed the first year of my PhD and was too busy learning how to tease apart molecules to give diagnosis much thought. Besides, that was the province of medics, not scientists. I belonged to the crowd studying the brain from the inside looking out, not the outside looking in. But now, I wanted to know. I wanted to meet someone at the very beginning of their descent and understand how we first lock horns with the disease, and what this means to those as confused as I once was. I also wanted a closer look at how our present understanding of the disease was reached. What did my colleagues and other scientists think caused it? Where were we in terms of an effective treatment?

What follows is a critical and impassioned journey to answer such questions, and a look at the surprising human stories that gave us this deeper understanding. Sometimes I worried that my persistence might have got the better of me; that in undertaking this endeavour I was reminding my father of a painful time in his life. But it was okay, he said. Everyone should grow old like those expats – laughing, sipping tea, chatting about friends and family. Sharing our experience is how we get there.

4

Diagnosis

One loyal friend is worth ten thousand relatives.

Euripides, attributed

ONE MORNING IN late 2014 Arnold Levi, an eighty-two-year-old retired film director from South Africa, walked into his local doctor's clinic in London with his best friend's son, Danie. The pair had known each other for more than thirty years; Danie's father had grown up with Arnold at a boarding school on the outskirts of Johannesburg. Arnold was sent away to school at the age of five, and he and Danie's father had instantly bonded. 'My dad was one of three brothers,' Danie told me. 'I think Arnold loved him because they protected him at school. They treated him like family.'

Something had been wrong with Arnold for nearly a year. In December 2013 Danie noticed some unsettling changes in his behaviour. Intelligent, self-reliant and streetwise, Arnold almost never had any trouble navigating the London Underground; every few months he would get the Tube from his home in west London and travel into the city to meet Danie for dinner.

But things began to change. Arnold seemed increasingly distressed by the journey, Danie recalled. One day, when they met outside the station, he appeared 'flustered', 'agitated', 'cross'. It wasn't like him, said Danie.

When Arnold was twenty, he moved to London to pursue his dream of becoming an actor. He played small parts in several films but soon changed tack when a colleague asked him for help teaching singers how to act. Arnold agreed, and enjoyed a fine career directing thereafter. He never married and had no children, but always stayed in touch with his childhood friend back in Johannesburg. Twenty years later, Danie moved to London for work as a stockbroker. 'When I moved here I lived close to Arnold, and he always watched out for me. "If you ever need a place to stay," he'd say, "you can always stay with me." I always knew that support was there.' As Arnold got older, Danie watched over his father's old friend in the same way.

In the months leading up to that day on the Tube, Danie began to spot problems with Arnold's memory. At first they seemed minor: he forgot his passport for a flight to New York, for example; he forgot that Danie had been on holiday. Typical things. But something about their frequency and nature felt atypical. Only in retrospect is Arnold's experience unsurprising. During the incipient phase of Alzheimer's symptoms, it is just about impossible to know that such lapses indicate the disease. 'My memory's shocking,' Danie told me. 'Literally, I can't remember what I did on the weekend. I just don't have the bandwidth to retain it. So when somebody else doesn't remember something you're not particularly surprised. But it was these little situations that just . . . jarred. They weren't normal. They didn't sit right.'

Danie arranged a private car to collect Arnold for their next outing. But when the driver arrived at the house, Arnold wasn't in. The driver called Danie, who then called Arnold. No answer. Earlier in the week, when Danie rang to arrange the lunch, he remembered that Arnold had kept misunderstanding the instruction and thought he was supposed to meet Danie where he used to work – a studio in north London. 'I said, "No no, the driver's gonna pick you, so don't go anywhere, yeah?" But he just kept on. I was thinking, what is it about the bloody . . .? Just stay at home! You don't have to do anything! You'll just be delivered here. What's wrong with you!?' Danie tried calling the house an hour later. Again, no answer. Now he was getting worried. He called the studio – Arnold was there.

It turned out he'd had no memory of ever discussing being collected by a private car. Danie told him not to worry, and asked if he felt comfortable getting a cab to the right location. He did, and so Danie, somewhat relieved, tried to put the mishap down as another harmless 'senior moment'.

His relief was short-lived – Arnold didn't arrive. Two hours later, he rang Danie from home. 'He called me and said, "Listen, I'm sorry, I don't know what happened . . . I think I've had a turn . . . I didn't know where I was . . . But I came across a Tube station and got myself home."' Later, Danie discovered that Arnold had forgotten what to do after leaving the studio and, confused, had then spent the time aimlessly wandering around the city. At that point, the young South African knew that he needed to take him to a doctor.

As they walked through the corridors of the Richford Gate medical practice – a wide, three-storey, sand-brick building occupying a quiet residential street in west London – a German physician called Jens Foell greeted them. Unexpectedly, Arnold introduced Danie as 'Mathew', Arnold's neighbour. They laughed it off, and went to take a seat in Foell's office. Already suspecting what might be wrong, Foell politely asked how he could be of assistance.

So Arnold said, 'Well, it's Mathew—'

'No, Arnold,' Danie interrupted, 'it's me, *Danie*.'

Arnold continued: 'He's been having some trouble.'

There was a momentary silence – and Foell, now unsure which of the two men was the patient, looked towards Danie.

'Arnold,' said Danie, 'we're here for *you*.'

'Oh really?' Arnold replied. 'I had no idea.'

In August 2015 I caught the London Underground to Arnold's house in Notting Hill, with a bag of fresh grapes and a box of Swiss chocolates. It was a warm, cloudy afternoon, with streets full of people eating lunch alfresco, hoping to see the sun. I had first heard of Arnold several months earlier through a medical colleague.

I'd asked if he knew any newly diagnosed patients willing to share their story. I wanted a classic case, I'd said – unaware then just how frail the term 'classic' is for Alzheimer's – and he'd responded by providing Danie's phone number. When I then called Danie, he was keen to talk to me. He said he felt alone.

Before entering Arnold's home, Danie briefed me outside. He had explained to Arnold who I was and why I was visiting – although he had to admit the likelihood that Arnold really remembered was slim.

We rang the doorbell. For a minute no sound emanated from the house, and, it being a holiday weekend, Danie feared Arnold might have wandered off somewhere unchaperoned. A moment later, however, the door opened and I was introduced to Arnold. He had curly white hair, glacier-blue eyes, and a broad, unabashed smile that instantly put one at ease. He was thin and willowy, casually yet smartly dressed in a dark purple shirt, check shorts and pointed leather shoes. He offered me a drink, which I politely refused, and the three of us sat down in a sitting room off the kitchen.

Ceiling-high windows flooded the room with natural light, Middle Eastern rugs blanketed the floor, old wooden dressers held ornate antique statues, and eighteenth-century artwork hung from every wall. Works on Mozart, Michelangelo and Wagner filled his bookshelves, as well as titles by Dickens and G. A. Henty. Here lived a man utterly devoted to learning, I thought. How cruel it was that this too would soon be taken from him; a love of books and knowledge made it all the more painful to lose one's memory. And beside me, arranged on his desk, were framed black and white photographs of his parents, and Danie's father, in Johannesburg. It was like stepping into a time capsule whose keeper has left a small simulacrum of himself.

We started talking. He spoke slowly, his voice low and sonorous, with an acquired English accent poles apart from Danie's clipped South African twang. I asked him questions about his life and friendship with Danie and his father. I asked him about his career, and the stories behind some of the beautiful objects surrounding us. His answers were eloquent and enlightened; he was clearly a highly intelligent man. Indeed, if we'd kept with this line of conversation I wouldn't have noticed anything was amiss. I then began asking him about the present. What were his neighbours like? Did he have friends living nearby? This is where things started to unravel.

'It's funny you should ask that,' Arnold said, 'because that was during the war . . . but I don't like going down this road.'

I changed topic and asked what he liked to do during the day, now that he was retired.

'I had to look after my mother and sister . . . this was during the war of course . . . but that isn't a very fit subject.'

Danie chimed in: 'Arnold, I think what Joseph was actually asking you was what do you like doing *today*.'

'Oh yes, of course, my apologies. Well, I was always very keen to live on my own. I couldn't wait to get out [of South Africa] . . . and don't forget, it was the end of the war . . . I would offer you something to drink but I don't think I'm going to.'

'Why not?' asked Danie.

'Well . . . I don't really know.'

The contrast between Arnold's awareness of the past, of memories far away in space and time, and his ability to make sense of the present was staggering. Danie had coaxed him several times into trying to answer some of my questions more accurately, offering gentle help here and there. But there was no denying it: Arnold was fading. The disease had taken its first casualty, a brain region right next to the hippocampus known as the parahippocampal gyrus. This is where new memories are stored and retrieved. It's why short-term memory loss is the first symptom of Alzheimer's. It provides a kind of memory pit stop, so that memories can be processed and then eventually transferred to the frontal cortex for long-term storage. We don't know why this region is targeted first. Plaques and tangles will ultimately invade other parts of Arnold's brain, including the frontal cortex, but for now, those appear mercifully intact.

'Shall I give you the tour?' Arnold asked me. We'd been talking in his sitting room for about half an hour, during which I'd also noticed his mirthful, tongue-in-cheek sense of humour. He'd often playfully reproach Danie for not remembering something, or if he suspected Danie was being mischievous behind his back. 'Don't play that game with me, young man!' he'd admonish.

Arnold then took us to see his attic. According to Danie, this is where he spends most of his time. It looked much like the sitting room, only with more books and bigger paintings. Danie was particularly keen to see it today, to assess the recent water damage in the roof – patches of damp had slowly been creeping their way along the ceiling's coving, causing it to bow precariously above Arnold's photograph-laden dressers. In the adjacent bathroom, parts of the ceiling had collapsed altogether.

'Arnold! I'm gonna chase up that builder again!' Danie called from the bathroom. 'We really need to get this sorted!'

Arnold had weekly visits from NHS carers. I asked him what he thought of them.

'Carers?' he said, puzzled. 'Oh no . . . I don't know anything about that.'

'What about Tom?' reminded Danie, who was now busily inspecting the cornices above us. 'You know, that guy who comes round.'

'Tom? Tom . . . Oh yes . . . he's a pleasant man . . . probably at *least* twenty years younger than me though.'

While Danie continued to examine the ceiling, Arnold and I walked out on to a small balcony that overlooked a row of modest square gardens lining the street. The sky was still overcast. He pointed out a tall ash tree. 'That's my favourite tree on this road,' he said. 'It's beautiful. Do you see how it's actually two trees?' A second, darker tree was growing alongside it. And then, eyes still fixed on it, he said something unexpected: 'I have a lot of memories that mean a great deal to me . . . It worries me . . . But what can I do?' Then he looked at me with a shrug of resignation and added, 'Not a lot.'

I wondered what to make of Arnold's comments. Until that moment I'd only been able to talk to friends and carers about the condition; my granddad had already lost awareness of his memory problems when he visited us again from Iran. Perhaps the cruellest irony of Alzheimer's, for the family above all else, is that the more advanced it gets, the less cognisant a patient becomes of their plight. Arnold's moment of clarity was therefore all the more important, and a part of me wanted to press him for further insight.

But as we headed back downstairs, he quickly forgot what he'd said and asked me to remind him who I was. I told him I was a friend of Danie, and that I was writing a book on memory.

'Oh! Wonderful!' he exclaimed. 'But . . . I have to say, I don't think Danie will be much help for *that*.'

Arnold is in the early, mild stage of the disease, Dr Foell told me during our conversation in his office. Foell is a plain-speaking, eccentric physician. He immigrated to England shortly after the collapse of the Berlin Wall and has been a general practitioner for the past thirteen years. A shade under six foot, he's an astonishingly fit man who sits on an inflatable exercise ball during consultations and adopts a no-nonsense, almost predatory approach to solving his patients' problems. I liked him immediately.

It had been several weeks since I visited Arnold, and I wanted to learn more about how someone with Alzheimer's is diagnosed.

'Good question,' Foell admitted. 'I often say that the best way to find out would be to kill you, and then slice your brain to look for plaques and tangles. But that doesn't really help you!' The reality, Foell explained, is that diagnosis is not a single act; it's a process.

First, Arnold must be excluded from the range of other maladies causing memory loss – such as depression, infection, stroke and cancer. This is done by gathering a medical history, performing an examination and arranging blood tests. Then Foell needs to know that Arnold is safe. He needs to make sure nothing can happen to Arnold before their next meeting. He asks questions like 'Where have you been?', 'What did you do?', 'How do you look after yourself?', 'Can you talk me through a normal day?', 'Do you lock yourself out of the house?', 'Do you leave the cooking hob on?'

'I found it very disturbing that Arnold lived on his own,' Foell solemnly confessed. 'Without his friend's son, organising his safety wouldn't be possible.'

Globally, there's a new diagnosis every four seconds, and even that's a conservative estimate.[1] In England, for example, it's thought that only 48 per cent of people with dementia receive a diagnosis.[2] The remaining 52 per cent may be people whose symptoms are mistaken for something else – like stress, the side effects of medication, normal ageing – or elderly people who live alone. Isolated patients can go for years without a diagnosis because no one flags up that there's a problem. One has to wonder how many souls in total go undiagnosed; a recent estimate put the figure at 28 million.[3] This is clearly an enormous problem, but as we shall see in chapter eight, it's slowly being solved.

After Foell was satisfied that Arnold's circumstances presented no looming danger, he sent him to a remarkable modern creation known as a memory clinic.

'Lemon. Key. Ball.' *Lemon, key, ball. Lemon, key, ball.* I repeated the words over and over in my head, as if trying to put a paperweight on the memory. I'm doing the Addenbrooke's Cognitive Examination, or ACE, in the office of Karen Magorrian, a senior nurse at the Charing Cross Hospital Memory Clinic in west London. It was here – with her – that Arnold began his journey into Alzheimer's in earnest, and I wanted to retrace his steps as best I could.

'If I gave you a hundred, could you take away seven?' Karen had a distinctly soothing quality to her voice – an effect born out of twenty years' experience with dementia patients.

'Yes,' I replied.

'And what would your answer be?'

'Ninety-three.'

'Carry on please.'

'Eighty-six. Seventy-nine. Seventy-two. Sixty-five—'

'Lovely. Thank you. And what were those three words I asked you to remember?'

'Lemon, key, ball.'

'Good. Now I'm going to give you a name and address to remember: Harry Barnes, 73 Orchard Close, Kingsbridge, Devon.'

Bloody hell! 'Okay.'

'Can you repeat it?'

'Harry Barnes, 73, Orchard . . . Devon.'

'Try again.'

'Harry Barnes, 73, Orchard Close, Kings . . . *bridge*? Devon.'

'Lovely. Excellent.'

'Can you tell me the name of our current Prime Minister?'

'David Cameron.'

'And who was the female Prime Minister we once had?'

'Margaret Thatcher.' She must have had this kind of test, I thought, having suffered dementia in her final years.

Karen continued in this vein, going on to test areas of attention and visual-spatial cognition. She asked me to draw a clock, and identify pictures of animals and partially concealed letters. I scored ninety-three out of a hundred.

Embarrassingly, I fell short on the vocabulary section of the test. Karen asked me to name as many words as I could — no names or places — beginning with the letter P. After 'pen', 'pencil', 'paper' and 'pigeon', I threw in some fancy ones — 'palpable', 'polymath', 'perspicacious'. I managed a few more and then went completely blank. I was so nervous about the high expectations (I am writing a book, after all) that my brain just froze. Worse still, I started thinking about names and places — Peter, Peru, Patagonia — as if getting those out of the way would somehow help me find what was actually being asked of me. This section represented a tiny fraction of the test. I wondered what it would feel like to brain-freeze on every section, as many patients did. But *un*thinking my thoughts, unwinding my reason, reversing it all into a foggy, unreachable abstraction, was unimaginable. By definition, no clear-headed individual could understand what it felt like.

The purpose of a test like this isn't to provide a diagnosis, but rather to get some sense of a person's memory and thinking abilities. Memorising three words or an address, for example, are good ways of assessing working memory: a type of short-term memory that we use to carry out tasks. Recalling historical facts or animal names measures declarative memory: the form of long-term memory for knowledge and ideas gathered over a lifetime (discussed in chapter three). The more active parts of the test – drawing a clock, summoning maths and vocabulary skills – determine what's known as executive function: the cognitive processes we use to achieve a certain goal.

Karen then explained what happens to a decidedly poor scorer. A group of neurologists, psychiatrists and nurses will meet for a *House*-style brainstorming session about what the diagnosis could be. The demands of the test can give an idea of what brain region is damaged, and if the patient seems depressed, stressed, or anxious, psychiatric problems are also considered. But if – like Arnold – the patient is elderly and displays a global failure of memory and cognition, Alzheimer's becomes the prime suspect. When brain scans corroborate that suspicion – showing cell loss beyond normal ageing, especially in the hippocampus – and further memory tests confirm it, 'probable Alzheimer's' is diagnosed, care is arranged, and acetylcholinesterase inhibitors are prescribed. And that's that. Treatment-wise, we're still where we were in the 1980s. 'We use Aricept [donepezil] a lot, and I'd say that in about 60 per cent of patients we get two or three years of stability. Their relatives will come back and tell us they are less agitated, and sleeping better. But some people just don't respond to it.'

Arnold was one of those people. By early 2016, just over two years since Danie first noticed his symptoms, Arnold continued to decline. His confusion was now verging on distress. He seemed frailer, less steady on his feet, almost 'shrunken', as Danie put it. He was also forgetting to feed himself, and increasingly relied on carers to prepare meals and deal with household affairs.

To a neurologist, this timeline is unsurprising: upon diagnosis, the average life expectancy is eight years, with most of that time spent in the moderate stage of the disease – what Arnold was now experiencing. To a neuroscientist, it suggests that plaques and tangles have finally infiltrated other parts of Arnold's brain, including the frontal lobes, destroying his ability to process logical thoughts, and the temporal and parietal lobes, giving rise to fear and anxiety. Because the temporal and parietal lobes process sensory information, damage can also result in paranoid delusions. A familiar person might seem like a stranger with bad intent, and relatives often recall moments when their loved one greets them with suspicious stares or hostility.

Lacking traditional family support, Arnold was beginning to become a danger to himself. One day, the carers arrived to discover that he had left all the cooker hobs on, filling the house with gas. On another, they found bruises running up his arm; it turned out he'd fallen down the stairs in the middle of the night. Determined to make life as comfortable as possible, Danie arranged private care for Arnold and juggled his own work–life commitments by requesting daily reports from the new carers.

Danie's father flew over from South Africa, and used the time with his old friend to recount stories from their childhood in Johannesburg. Arnold listened with a mixture of mirth and bewilderment. For Danie's father, the friend he knew was still there, despite everything.

But it wasn't long before what Arnold's adopted family feared most happened. When Danie met Arnold at the memory clinic for a follow-up appointment, he was greeted as a complete stranger. 'I could have been anybody, a passer-by in the street,' Danie said in a lugubrious voice when I met him for coffee. We were sitting in a small café in Mayfair, where he works, on a clear spring morning. 'I told him my name to help jog his memory, and he did sort of recognise me. He knows he knows me, but he can't remember how he knows me.'

I asked Danie how things were at home. 'Oh God. It's like

dealing with a child,' he confessed. 'We had this whole saga about the kettle, because I took away his stove-top kettle and bought him an electric kettle. Well, that just blew his mind! He didn't want to use it. So it eventually disappeared and I had to buy another one – we've been through several kettles now. I bought him a new bedside lamp, and a few weeks later *that* disappeared. It's like they're intruders into his world.

'I bought him a toaster at the weekend and just put it on the counter and started using it, because if I have a conversation with him about it, I'm gonna want to strangle myself *and* him. I've got to think about my sanity, too.'

Danie had no burning desire to put Arnold in a nursing home, but things were falling apart. To test the waters, he took Arnold to visit one that had been recommended by a friend. It was privately run, and was also near Arnold's house. The facility had two dementia wings, catering for both moderate- and late-stage Alzheimer's. 'This is fascinating,' Arnold said as the pair were shown around. In the moderate wing, he was his usual cheerful self. He shook hands and exchanged pleasantries with the residents, gazing in astonishment like a tourist visiting a zoo, said Danie, who, in stark contrast, was horrified by what he saw. 'I hated it,' he admitted. 'The people running it were really nice, but the residents, mostly women, all looked completely zonked out. I thought, *Well, you're definitely not at this stage. I can't put you here.*'

The pair then walked into the late-stage wing. The rooms were spacious and well decorated, and it had a calming, serene atmosphere. Nevertheless, the residents' state of mind couldn't be ignored. Hearing Danie recall this part of their trip, an image of my grandfather flashed into my mind. Towards the end, he remained slouched in a chair, silent but for the occasional wail for his long-deceased wife – a shell of his former self. Late-stage Alzheimer's has been described as 'death before death'. By this point, the disease has systematically wiped out huge chunks of brain tissue, effectively erasing the ability to speak, eat, swallow and even smile. A late-stage patient needs care twenty-four hours a day, with everything, from getting dressed to walking to the bathroom. They are utterly dependent on others; left alone, they will spend the entire day staring into space before dying of starvation or an infection.

The tragedy wasn't lost on Arnold. In this wing, he was much less sanguine. 'Oh dear,' he groaned, disturbed by what he was seeing. 'I certainly don't want this to happen to *me*.' Danie thanked the staff for their time, and promptly took his old companion home.

Though he had thought that moving Arnold was the right approach, after the visit to the care home he vowed to rededicate himself to Arnold's care. He was going to keep Arnold at home for as long as the illness permitted. 'It's hard. It's really hard. You're expected to have all the answers, and I *don't* have all the answers. There are nights when I work until eight o'clock and then rush over to make sure he's all right. I'll end up getting home and eating dinner at ten. But these are my weak moments; otherwise I'm really happy to do it.'

I had long wondered what patients do when they have no family. Apart from emotional support, family members take care of the minutiae of everyday life. Although hired carers can do this to an extent, they were certainly no substitute for my grandfather's three daughters, who had stayed in Iran after my father and uncle left to learn English and get a decent education. In his final years, my aunts fed and washed him, did his shopping, managed his estate, and spent countless hours – however futile – exploring photograph albums with him, explaining each picture of the family and life he had once had. This is the power of family. They thread everything together; they keep things on an even keel.

Arnold may not have the same level of support, but in Danie he has one astonishingly loyal friend. I made a point of visiting Arnold again a few months later. Despite not responding to current treatment, this charming octogenarian has helped make physicians, memory specialists and scientists alike more aware of how dementia manifests in the real world. While much attention in novels and popular film is given to early-onset Alzheimer's, the reality is that most patients are elderly people like Arnold. His story is one of millions whose ending we must change. To do that, scientists know that an effective treatment can only come from a better understanding of the disease. And this will only come from the burgeoning field of medical genetics.

5

The Alzheimer's Gene

I can't think. But I still feel. And most of the time I feel scared.
Scared because it's too soon. I haven't finished yet.

Nicola Wilson, *Plaques and Tangles*

THREE AUNTS, ONE uncle and now her father. With that,
Carol Jennings, a thirty-year-old teacher from Nottingham,
had made up her mind. On 11 April 1986 she walked to
her desk, took out a sheet of Basildon Bond paper, and began.

'Dear Sir,' she penned in dark blue ink. 'I was very interested
to read of your research in the *Alzheimer's Disease Society News* and
think my family could be of use.' On a separate sheet Carol jotted
down a family tree depicting relatives from both her father's generation and grandfather's generation. 'Actually, I am the daughter of
Walter,' she continued, 'who you will see from the family tree is
sixty-three years old and has Alzheimer's, as does his sister, Audrey.
His brother, Arthur, may also have the disease . . . please contact
me at the above address if you think we could be of help.'

The letter was addressed to St Mary's Hospital in London, where
a group of researchers were chasing a lead many considered a long
shot: could Alzheimer's be genetic?

This radical idea had started to gain traction when Leonard
Heston, a physician in Minnesota, published some astonishing observations in October 1981.[1] Using brain samples from over 2,000
post-mortems done in Minnesota state hospitals, he'd found that
relatives of middle-aged, or 'early-onset', Alzheimer's patients were

more likely to develop the disease when they reached middle age themselves. Even those with self-confessed ignorance of genetics knew this had the earmarks of inheritance; indeed, Heston wasn't the first to suggest the link: physicians in Sweden and Switzerland during the 1950s spotted the trend while looking through hospital records of families with a history of dementia. At that time, however, genes were thought to be entities that only gave rise to basic aspects of human biology such as height, build and eye colour. They certainly weren't believed to have much (if anything) to do with the intricate vagaries of the mind. In any case, genes were still inaccessible molecules and so physicians were more interested in the chemical basis of disease.

But by the 1980s the DNA double helix had come and gone and gene sequencing technology was well on its way. George Glenner, a molecular pathologist at the US National Institute on Aging, seized upon Heston's results.

Quiet and reserved, formal and aloof, with wavy silver hair and an unassuming gaze, Glenner didn't know much about the brain when he began working on Alzheimer's in 1983. He was considered an outsider by many neuroscientists. After training at Johns Hopkins University he quickly became fascinated by how diseases develop at the cellular level, and therefore chose to specialise in pathology. In particular, Glenner was puzzled by amyloid – which he called 'one hell of a nasty substance'[2] – and soon became hell-bent on figuring out what it really was.

Glenner's mission epitomised the confidence that targeting the plaques was medicine's best bet. No one actually knew if they caused the disease, nor whether they formed before or after neurons started dying. And no one knew if they were more or less culpable than the tangles seen inside neurons. Nevertheless, their lingering presence demanded answers; *disproving* their significance became just as imperative as proving it. With access to freezers filled with donated brains – one of the first Alzheimer's 'brain banks' – Glenner set to work, mechanically slicing and grinding up each one, uprooting blood vessels, sifting out connective tissue, and chemically pulverising what was left until nothing but amyloid remained. After a year – in May 1984 – he'd finally managed to extract the protein that formed the plaques' core, and dubbed it beta-amyloid, a term that would resonate among neuroscientists for the next thirty years.[3]

Glenner then performed a quantum leap. In Heston's study it had been noted that many Alzheimer's patients' relatives had a high incidence of Down's syndrome in the family. Doctors were realising, moreover, that nearly everyone with Down's syndrome who reached middle age invariably died with a dementia uncannily similar to Alzheimer's. The conditions clearly had some sort of connection, but what was it?

Down's syndrome, a genetic condition that develops from an abnormal extra copy of chromosome 21, was the only other known condition where vast deposits of amyloid saturate the brain. And when Glenner began examining amyloid from Down's syndrome patients, he realised it was made up of the same protein found in the brains of Alzheimer's patients.[4] This suggested something wholly unexpected. Maybe, for some people, there was a *gene* for Alzheimer's – lurking somewhere inside chromosome 21.

And so as soon as Glenner's results were released, scientists started gathering DNA samples from families showing signs of an inherited form of Alzheimer's, which they called 'familial' Alzheimer's disease. One sample came from a large family of Canadians of British origin, whose ancestors emigrated to Canada in 1837; in just eight generations a whopping fifty-four cases of Alzheimer's had been reported. A German family had twenty cases in six generations. A Russian family showed twenty-three cases in six generations. A large Italian family, whose members had branched out to France and the US, had forty-eight cases in eight generations.

Familial Alzheimer's looked identical to the more common, non-inherited version; the only noteworthy difference was the age of onset: its symptoms appeared much sooner, usually in people's fifties, forties and even late thirties. The discovery of familial Alzheimer's was revolutionary not only because it proved Alzheimer's could be genetic, but because its genetic origin offered scientists the first real clue as to how the predominant, late-onset disease manifested. With a gene as their starting point scientists could investigate what other molecules it interacted with, and thereby begin to stich together a biochemical web of causation. It was akin to pinning a photograph of a Mafioso on a drawing board for detectives then to map out the entire crime syndicate.

By 1986, acting on Glenner's findings, several US groups successfully decoded the DNA sequence of beta-amyloid.[5] They christened the gene APP (for amyloid precursor protein). That gave the scientists-cum-detectives a suspect. But APP by itself wasn't enough. They needed to learn if the gene was guilty by finding out if it had been permanently altered from what was normal. And for that, they needed to find a mutation.

Tall and brunette, with thin, sparrow-like features and narrow, enquiring eyes, Carol Jennings was an extremely conscientious woman who knew a problem when she saw one. Her father, Walter, was the eldest of fifteen children born into a working-class Protestant family. A milkman who'd served in the navy during the war, Walter was a scrupulous man who worked hard to look after Carol, the apple of his eye. He was known for his chatty, high-spirited temperament and the thorough way he managed the family's finances, constantly writing things down and chasing up monthly dues from the Nottingham Co-op.

By his fifty-eighth birthday, however, Walter was becoming 'a different person' – quiet, disengaged and strangely no longer able to organise his accounts. Sometimes he seemed genuinely befuddled by even the most routine of tasks: while shopping he would often pick up the wrong things and then put them in somebody else's trolley. When the family took him to a doctor they were told he had dementia, probably Alzheimer's. There was no discussion about a cause or even his disproportionate age.

But Walter was not the only one: four of his younger siblings started experiencing symptoms as they approached sixty themselves. Ironically, because lots of the family were getting Alzheimer's this early, many of them thought it was quite normal. But not Carol, whose letter soon found its way to St Mary's Hospital. And there, working in a laboratory, was a twenty-eight-year-old molecular geneticist named Alison Goate.

Goate was part of a large group searching for Alzheimer's mutations. 'Everybody acknowledged that there were these families with Alzheimer's that appeared to be genetic,' she told me in her lilting, transatlantic accent during a call from New York, where she now works as director of the Mount Sinai Alzheimer's Research Center. 'But these families were extremely rare, so people didn't really talk about genes for Alzheimer's at the time.'

Energised by Carol's story, St Mary's immediately responded saying they wanted to know more. They arranged for doctors to ask questions and collect blood samples. And so Carol contacted the entire family, asking them all to meet at her house to donate samples and tell the doctors everything they knew. 'I was always impressed by Carol,' Goate said. 'She was like a cheerleader the way she persuaded family members to participate.'

Back in London, the hunt for the gene mutation was on. It relied on exploiting a key principle of genetics: genes that sit close to one another on a chromosome tend to be inherited together – they are said be genetically linked. This meant that if certain chunks of DNA were always seen in a family with a history of dementia, one could infer that a mutation was hiding somewhere in that region of DNA. If the proverbial DNA search engine worked, it promised a new era of personalised medicine. Treatments targeting a genetic defect could conceivably fix the problem's root cause, blowing drugs like tacrine out of the water. 'The acetylcholine drugs are approved because there's nothing else,' Goate said. 'They may be better than nothing for some people, but they're treating the symptoms rather than the cause. But your genetic predisposition might suggest which drugs you should be taking.'

Still, finding a mutation wasn't easy. Although DNA is a simple molecule of four repeating chemical groups – Adenine (A), Thymine (T), Cytosine (C) and Guanine (G) – its code is 3 billion letters long in humans. Written out, it would amount to 200 volumes each 1,000 pages long, which would take a typist grinding eight hours a day half a century to complete. How could anyone expect to find a spelling mistake in that? Fortunately, the Down's syndrome connection and the whereabouts of the APP gene gave Goate a good place to start: chromosome 21.

Just four years later, in February 1991, Goate found the mutation.[6] It was a single letter of DNA code – a 'T' that should have been a 'C'. Three billion letters and that's all it took to dismantle Carol's family. If there's any field that makes one truly appreciate the knife-edge we live on, genetics is surely it.

The discovery provoked a blizzard of media attention. FAMILY LINK OFFERS HOPE OF ALZHEIMER'S DISEASE CURE, declared *The Times*. GENE MUTATION THAT CAUSES ALZHEIMER'S IS FOUND, hailed the *New York Times*.

In the wake of the discovery, Goate and some colleagues visited Carol and her family in Nottingham, where they had all congregated in Carol's living room. They were eager to know what had been found and what it actually meant for them. Goate explained that the mutation is what geneticists call fully penetrant: anyone who carries it will definitely develop early-onset Alzheimer's. It was also dominant, meaning they all had a 50 per cent chance of carrying it. Then came the crux: there was a test. Anyone who wanted to know could do so, including Carol. Both choices were reasonable. Knowing meant she would be free of worry were the test negative, or could plan the rest of her life accordingly were it positive. Then again, not knowing meant living without the burden of such knowledge were it positive.

There's a name for this kind of dilemma. It's called a 'Hobson's choice', after the sixteenth-century stable owner who had a stable of forty horses but only ever offered his customers the horse nearest the stable door. The choice is thus an illusion because only one option really exists, and you can take it or leave it. So, would you want to know?

There was a time, during my PhD, when I was offered the

chance to know if I would eventually develop Huntington's disease. A friend was studying it for her own thesis and was interested in how it affected blood. For this she needed blood from healthy volunteers, and I donated without fully realising she would, obviously, have to check that I really *was* a healthy volunteer. After the phlebotomist withdrew my blood I was handed a form asking if I wanted to be informed if it tested positive. Granted, the chances of me having it are next to zero; the condition is hereditary and no one in my family has ever had it.

But I still said no. Huntington's, like Alzheimer's, is a cruel and devastating condition. It causes erratic, uncontrolled movements and cognitive impairment that steadily descends into a nightmarish dementia all of its own. There is no cure or treatment in sight. And so the only thing worse than succumbing to the disorder, in my mind, was knowing I would succumb to it years beforehand.

Carol, too, said no. She didn't see the point in knowing when there was nothing she could do about it anyway. In August 2012, healthy but approaching her family's age of onset, she told a reporter: 'I never did want to know. Having the test has always been an option: I could find out now. But I think I would just collapse in a heap if I thought, "This was it."'[7] After Walter died she'd devoted thirty years to Alzheimer's awareness and research. Drug companies flew her around the world to give talks about what it was and how it affected her family. And every year she volunteered for brain scans, helping scientists amass an invaluable record. Because the research was always double-blinded, even the researchers remained oblivious to Carol's ambivalent genetic fate.

'My nan had *fifteen* kids. I mean, you can't even imagine that, can you?' Carol said, with a quiet laugh and a shake of her head. It was early in the afternoon of 18 September 2015. I was sitting in the living room of a modestly sized house on a narrow, leafy avenue in Coventry, England, talking to Carol and her husband, Stuart.

'I'm trying to think who else had it,' Stuart said, while handing me a cup of tea. He was fifty-nine years old, a university chaplain and historian, with deep-set eyes and a soft, cherubic face. 'Let's think, Carol. Your aunty Audrey had it. Your uncle had it. Kath's got it at the moment but I think that's age-related Alzheimer's.'

'Yes, oh yes,' said Carol, in a softly spoken voice freighted with compassion. 'And did you know, my nan had *fifteen* kids. You can't even imagine that, can you?'

Carol was diagnosed in December 2012. She was fifty-eight years old: the same age her father, Walter, started displaying symptoms. According to Stuart, there had been noticeable lapses in her memory and cognition since 2008. 'You can't live with somebody for thirty years and not notice slight, subtle changes.' Carol kept forgetting what she'd gone into a room for, he said. Then she began storing numerous items of clothing, inexplicably, beneath her pillow. They didn't seem like particularly serious mistakes at the time. 'Carol would say to me, "The trouble with you is that you're looking for it." But things weren't right.' At work Carol had become uncharacteristically disorganised, missing deadlines and forgetting to file paperwork. Again, little things. But that was just the start – a slow accrual, carrying her mind gently and irrevocably towards the baffling ailment that plagued her father.

While the three of us chatted, she pointed at a black and white picture of Walter resting on a nearby wooden cabinet. He had a thin, rugged face, wore thick rectangular glasses, and was neatly dressed in a white-striped shirt and tie. I asked if she remembered what made her write the letter to St Mary's all those years ago.

'There was *something* . . .' she mused, furrowing her brow. 'For a while things were going . . . a bit pear-shaped . . . there was *some* sort of thing, I'm sure, that was . . . a little bit . . . strange.'

As I sat there, listening intently, seeing how a slip in just one gene is expressed in the vicissitudes of personhood, I was struck by how acutely unaware of Alzheimer's Carol had become. Here, in front of me, was a woman who had transformed our understanding of the disease, a woman who had devoted most of her life to raising awareness of it. Now, she was scarcely able to say its name.

Then she chuckled. 'I mean, the family my nan had got, how many kids did they have? *Fifteen*, wasn't it?'

'Your grandma did, yeah,' Stuart replied. He said this in a calm, dispassionate way – not impatiently or patiently – just in the way he always spoke to his wife. He wasn't going to let the disease change that.

We finished our tea and went to have some lunch. We ate back in the comfort of the living room, exchanging anecdotes and shifting the conversation to jocularity, Carol naturally being fairly quiet but smiling just the same. Afterwards, she went upstairs to see her ninety-year-old mother, Joyce, who lived with the couple and was now, incredibly, helping care for Carol. Joyce was quite healthy for her age, according to Stuart, and of course knew all about the condition after caring for Walter thirty years earlier.

Now alone with Stuart, I asked him frankly: how was he coping? He explained how he teeters from stoicism to despair. He said he once knew a woman who got on a plane to Bern, Barcelona and Buenos Aires, a woman who travelled the world to speak at conferences to neuroscientists and the public. But now, he said, 'I wouldn't trust her to walk up the road to the grocery store.' Stuart is fighting to save Carol; every few months the couple make the trip to London to try the latest experimental treatment. But Carol is fading and he knows it.

'I think it's too late for Carol,' Stuart confessed. 'It's the kids we're fighting for now.'

A few weeks later I met John Jennings, the couple's thirty-year-old son, in his apartment amid the bewitching dark stone buildings of Edinburgh, Scotland. He was tall and thin, had dark brown eyes, and resembled Carol. An exceedingly thoughtful man with a quiet seriousness of purpose, John had become increasingly involved in raising awareness since his mother's decline. Her affliction is something he's all too familiar with, for he now faces the same terrifying odds she did.

'Because it's always been there it's a huge part of who I am,'

John said, recounting the media attention and intense scientific interest in his family during the early 1990s. As a child, he didn't think anything was particularly amiss with his grandfather. Walter was an old man as far as he was concerned; his affliction – whatever it was – was simply his way of dying. 'I remember visiting him in the ward. He would just sit in this huge padded chair.' John remembers seeing his mum, who was never good with needles, passed out on the couch after the St Mary's team took blood samples – including his. Only when John reached adulthood, however, did the profundity of his family's situation, and the stark decisions he would have to make, finally sink in.

Did he want the test? 'I've chosen not to know,' John confided in me with a philosophical tone. 'Because Mum always used to say, "You know, you could get hit by a bus," and part of the human condition is that you plan as though you're gonna live for ever. But I've sort of convinced myself that I have the gene, which is quite common to people from these families; we assume we have it, and if it turns out we don't it will be a bonus.

'And because I've had so long to build a way of dealing with it, I don't have the all-gripping fear that a lot of people have. Even though Mum was really upset when she first had something resembling a diagnosis, she's happy enough at the moment. So, from her perspective, it's sort of . . . okay.'

As anyone would be, John's now keen to discover where the mutation came from. Carol's great-grandmother, a woman born in 1861 – just a few years shy of Alzheimer himself – was the earliest known carrier, he explained. But more than anything, he wants to know what his ancestors' lives were like. He's amazed at how the family's symptoms are being re-enacted with an almost hallucinatory quality: at Carol's wedding, for example, Walter got confused and told people that his daughter was getting married soon – Carol did the same thing at her daughter's wedding; and Walter often followed Joyce around the house – which, according to Stuart, is now exactly what Carol does as well.

John then switched on his laptop to show me a Facebook group for other people confronted by early-onset dementia. One conversation thread described a single mother who'd recently tested positive and was wrestling with the decision whether to tell her fifteen-year-old son. Another told of three young siblings, two of whom possess a mutation that will initiate the disease in their late thirties. John replies to them all; the crucial thing, he says, is to keep talking about it.

When I asked John how much he talked to his own family about it, and what those conversations were even like, he gave me a wry smile and laughed. 'We've actually got this middle-class British problem of not talking about anything of any kind of emotional import. We still do that; we'll skirt around the issue. Even if something comes on the news about dementia, we'll watch it in silence and then discuss what comes on afterwards.

'We did once speak about what it would be like,' he offered, recollecting a wine-fuelled evening while on holiday with his parents some years earlier. 'We said that it would be like watching a television screen and the static slowly increasing.'

Confronted by a 50 per cent chance of that analogy eventually becoming reality, how much did he think about it? 'More or less every day,' he admitted. 'I wake up in the night sometimes and think about it. But then I'll think about the fact that we're losing Mum, which is a weird kind of grieving process, losing somebody over a long period of time. And then I feel guilty because it's something she's experiencing and I'm just worrying about. So there's a lot of different ways it enters your consciousness.'

On the plane back to London I tried to make sense of Carol's story. A spate of unanswerable questions filled my head. How would I feel if my grandfather's Alzheimer's was familial? Would I have said 'no' to that test? What if John had changed his mind and learned he was positive before Carol got sick? Would her right not to know have obliged him to secrecy? Could you even keep something like that from your parents? And what did this form of Alzheimer's say about human existence? Are we prisoners of our genes?

Then I remembered something Stuart had said to me just before I left their home. 'If we were to have a poem that encapsulated our way of thinking about this, it would be Dylan Thomas's "Do Not go Gentle into that Good Night". Because we're not giving up. And all the research and the press . . . well, it's just our way of saying, "*Fuck you*, we're having the last word."'

And they will. Recognised as the first discovered cause of Alzheimer's, the APP mutation gave scientists the evidence they desperately needed. No longer did they have to guess if amyloid was responsible, now they had tangible proof. There was still much work to be done: scientific discoveries generally take about twenty years to ascend the throne of clinical and commercial use. That time would be filled sketching separate but no less urgent explanations, such as how tangles fit into all this, and whether a medicine based on APP would help people with non-genetic, late-onset Alzheimer's. But there was no doubt, the field had moved up a gear. Today, thousands of scientific papers have been published as a result; each one a small, incremental discovery bringing us closer to a cure; and each made possible because a curious milkman's daughter sat down to write a letter.

6

The Science Behind the Headlines

DEMENTIA AND ALZHEIMER'S LEADING CAUSE OF DEATH IN
ENGLAND AND WALES

Guardian headline, November 2016

AND THERE IT was. Confirmation of what many had feared. The headline reached numerous broadcasts and, thanks to colleagues, appeared numerous times in my inbox, like an alarm I couldn't switch off. Alzheimer's had now overtaken heart disease as a leading cause of death in my country and one of its closest neighbours. Citing a report by the Office for National Statistics, the author quoted an increase from 13.4 per cent of all recorded deaths in 2014 to 15.2 per cent in 2015.[1]

Reading the article, I was torn: as a patient relative, I felt sorrow but also relief: *That's terrible, though maybe now people will do more about it.* As a scientist, both emotions yielded to anger: *It should not have got this bad!* Clearly an effective treatment was now urgent. Of course, not a week goes by when the news doesn't declare a breakthrough with the spectre of a cure. The irony is that the ceaseless headlines reflect how much we don't know, rather than how much we do.

People often ask me, 'What is Alzheimer's disease?' I respond with an explanation of plaques and tangles, cell death and memory loss. But by the end of the twentieth century, the real question was where did Alzheimer's come from? How did it start?

Three remarkable theories emerged and neuroscience adopted a new mantra: Alzheimer's disease is a *process*.

As a science obsessed with small changes occurring over long stretches of time, it seems apt that genetics would be the field to usher in this concept. The marriage of disciplines hatched a hybrid called neuro-genetics: a special branch of genetics focused solely on the brain. It also ushered in a new armada of neurogeneticists. Among them is John Hardy, the most cited Alzheimer's researcher in the UK. Hardy has been working on dementia since the days of Kidd and Terry, when only a handful of people on the planet were focusing their research efforts on the disease. An avuncular, plain-speaking man, he has an almost celebrity status among his peers, and is often seen wandering the corridors of his laboratory in University College London in shorts and flip-flops, a stack of papers under his arm, poking his head over the shoulders of young academics, eager to see what the new generation of researchers are up to.

In 1992 Hardy put forward a bold new theory on the cause of Alzheimer's, one that was to prove so alluring, so self-evident and so impressive in its scope that since then an explosion of work has emanated from it. 'In all cases of Alzheimer's disease,' he told me during my visit to his office, 'we have amyloid plaques scattered throughout the brain. In all cases we have tangles inside neurons. In all cases we have nerve cell loss. And in all cases we have a dementia. As scientists we have to work out which of those things is first. We have to put an *order* to them.'

And that's exactly what he did. Hardy argued that the formation of beta-amyloid plaques in the brain is the primary event in the disease. Tangles, neurotransmitter loss, cell death, memory loss and dementia, he said, are all secondary events – brain flotsam and jetsam left by a harrowing and crippling storm of amyloid. He called his theory the amyloid cascade hypothesis,[2] a hypothesis he confidently asserts is 'no question, the best idea'. He and his supporters are known as the Baptists (from Beta Amyloid Protein) – a highly appropriate name given the fervour of their belief in it.

Though beta-amyloid's function is still unknown, biochemists agree that it looks like a protein with responsibilities at the cell surface. Cell surface proteins often act like molecular drawbridges for the cell, permitting the entry and exit of other molecules. Alternatively, they can act as molecular antennae for communication with neighbouring cells. If one of these proteins malfunctions – due to a genetic mutation, say – the cell might self-destruct to stop the damage leaking into the cellular circuitry protecting us from cancer. At this level, life is ruthlessly totalitarian.

To play out Hardy's hypothesis, then, malfunctioning fragments of beta-amyloid first drift away from the neuron and accumulate as plaques. Over time, these plaques grow in size to the point where normal neuronal communication is no longer possible, like islands of waste preventing maritime trade. Starved of biochemical support, conditions inside the neuron start to break down – cue the tangles – and the neuron soon does what evolution has instructed it to do. It kills itself.

Exactly how beta-amyloid triggers such a neural catastrophe is, Hardy admits, a complete mystery. 'We don't know. I mean, we *really* don't know. And I would say that's the biggest hole. We just don't understand how plaques kill neurons.'

The theory had two key advantages. First, it put Alzheimer's disease on a temporal plane. Framing it this way meant scientists could make testable predictions about the disease's trajectory and evolution. Second, it gave drug companies another target to complement acetylcholine. The meagre effects of acetylcholine-based drugs created a dire need to try something new and left a gaping (and lucrative) hole for pharmaceutical companies to fill with new, amyloid-based therapeutics.

Families like the Jennings were a source of major support. 'Because we'd found families which had amyloid mutations,' Hardy explained, 'that told us that, in those families anyway, amyloid is where the disease starts. So the simplest thing to assume is that amyloid always starts it; that it's always the first event.'

Proof of Hardy's theory arrived when a group of researchers at

Athena Neurosciences, a San Francisco-based biotechnology company, did what was long considered impossible. On 9 February 1995 Athena's scientists injected mouse embryos with a human APP gene mutation.[3] The idea of a mouse possessing human DNA is too strange to contemplate. Suffice it to say, the invention broke new ground by providing a means to actually breed the disease ad infinitum.

So did these animals really get Alzheimer's? They certainly developed plaques in their brain, and showed cognitive impairments in memory-related tasks such as navigating a maze. But strangely, they didn't show any signs of tangles – nor, for that matter, a great deal of cell death. It was as if they had partial Alzheimer's. But the fact that Carol Jennings's mutation – a mutation leading to excessive beta-amyloid production – caused the animals' downfall provided strong evidence for Hardy's amyloid cascade hypothesis. It didn't prove the theory, but it might as well have, his supporters proclaimed. After all, no model is perfect. In an editorial in *Nature* the same year, Hardy boldly stated that the generation of amyloid plaques in these mice 'settles this argument, perhaps for good'.[4]

Working in Hardy's laboratory is an invigorating experience. In the years following my grandfather's diagnosis, reading scientific literature had left me awash with ifs, buts and maybes. Nearly everyone I told – family and friends alike – returned looks of soft commiseration: 'That's what happens when you get old,' they'd say over and over again. Working alongside Hardy, I felt grounded in my quest for a better answer.

But not everyone shares Hardy's conviction that beta-amyloid marks the start of Alzheimer's disease.

As dusk descended on a cool and clear April evening in 1984, Allen Roses, a neurologist at Duke University, North Carolina, waited anxiously at a railroad crossing, watching the cars of a passing coal train gently rattle by. The train was a rare sight. But of all the days it could appear, on that particular day it was most unwelcome. Standing next to him was a colleague, and in between them, lying on a wheeled stretcher, was an elderly woman with Alzheimer's, who had been pronounced dead only thirty minutes earlier. They were taking her from the hospital, down a narrow concrete track, to a post-mortem facility less than 300 yards away.

Roses didn't usually have to run an urban obstacle course as part of his day; his normal routine involved sitting at a lab bench. But that day was different. Roses' boss wanted him to head a new Alzheimer's research programme and so Roses submitted a grant application to the National Institute on Aging and was swiftly rejected. If Roses wanted the money, the NIA said, he would have to prove that he could get patient brain tissue from the hospital to the lab in less than one hour.

So as the train sluggishly rolled along the track, Roses and his colleague could do nothing but wait. When it finally passed, the pair dragged the stretcher the rest of the way as fast as they could. As they pushed through the doors to the post-mortem suite, they immediately checked their watches: forty-one minutes. They had done it.

Over the next few years Roses joined the hunt for an Alzheimer's gene, and by 1990 he had identified a genetic variant for late-onset Alzheimer's.[5] (Variants are not the same as mutations: whereas mutations often directly cause disease, variants simply increase a person's risk of disease. They are commonly dubbed 'genetic risk factors'.)

Meanwhile, one of Roses' colleagues, a neurologist named Warren Strittmatter, was busy trying to wrap his head around a perplexing technical issue with his experiments. Strittmatter, like George Glenner before him, was an amyloid expert. Whenever he purified amyloid from patient brains, however, he kept fishing out another protein stuck to the plaques. It must be a contaminant, he thought. But Roses wasn't so sure, and asked him to pursue the lead and identify the substance. Four months later Strittmatter discovered that it was apolipoprotein (APOE), a decidedly uninteresting liver protein that carries fat and cholesterol in the blood and can be found throughout the body. It probably had nothing to do with Alzheimer's.

But in that moment Roses had an epiphany. He knew the APOE gene was located on chromosome 19, the same chromosome in which his latest work had flagged up a new Alzheimer's gene. Was the connection mere coincidence? Roses didn't think so. His team, on the other hand, almost certainly did. They refused to do any more experiments on it, convinced, as Roses later put it, that 'the chief was off on one of his crazy ideas'.[6]

But Roses kept digging. He learned that the APOE gene exists in three versions – APOE2, APOE3 and APOE4 – and became struck by the possibility that one of these versions might increase the risk of late-onset Alzheimer's. The best way a version could be distinguished from the others was by a burgeoning technology called polymerase chain reaction (PCR). Invented in 1983 by the American biochemist Kary Mullis, PCR is essentially a DNA photocopier. It allows scientists to amplify tiny amounts of DNA for the purposes of paternity testing, forensics and medical diagnostics.

Although PCR is easy to perform, it helps to have an experienced hand. And so, ostracised by his team, Roses turned to his wife, Ann Saunders, a mouse geneticist well versed at PCR. By spring of 1992 the couple had unearthed a truly startling finding. APOE4 carriers have a high risk of developing both early- and late-onset Alzheimer's – fourfold higher if one copy of the gene is inherited, twelvefold with two copies. The gene is present in 30 per cent of the population and, astonishingly, in 50 per cent of all Alzheimer's patients, making it the leading genetic risk factor for the disease.[7]

But how could a liver protein be involved in Alzheimer's? At scientific conferences, where passions run high, the criticisms launched at Roses 'went from nasty to vicious', he recalled. But despite the scepticism, Roses persevered.

On 14 November 1995, at a debate over the motion 'This house believes beta-amyloid deposition causes Alzheimer's disease', he fired back. He presented a slideshow displaying three photographs. The first photograph was of a Japanese Shinto grave, an elaborate and complex work of art; the second was of an old tombstone found in a Catholic cemetery; the third was his father's grave, a bronze plaque in a Jewish cemetery. He pointed at them and said, 'Every one of these is absolutely diagnostic of what's underneath it. But nobody would say that the tombstone caused the death.'

But the analogy did little to dissuade the disbelievers. His intention, though, was not so much to dispel interest in beta-amyloid as it was to receive acknowledgement of APOE4. 'I have no doubt that there is plaque formation,' he assured me. 'I just don't think it's the cause. But everybody in the Alzheimer's community thought APOE4 was a big joke. They just didn't want to hear about it. I couldn't even get another grant to pursue it.'

Listening to Roses, I felt both sympathetic and inured to his plight. Scientists are not the paragons of mutual camaraderie we might imagine them to be – all hell-bent on uniting under one banner to seek the truth. They are human. Big intellects bring big egos, which partly explains why Roses was dismissed by so many. Although a string of European studies soon confirmed his discovery, by 1997 the Alzheimer's community was firmly focused on the amyloid cascade hypothesis. Unable to fund further work on APOE4, Roses was forced to leave academia and pursue the lead in the pharmaceutical industry. There, he pioneered a new theory on the cause of Alzheimer's, one that put APOE4 in the spotlight and which came to be called the mitochondrial-impairment hypothesis. Or more simply, 'type three diabetes'.

In type one diabetes, problems arise when the death of insulin-producing cells in the pancreas depletes the body of insulin. Type two diabetes, on the other hand, results from insulin resistance when cells stop responding to it following an excessive dietary intake of glucose (although genetic and lifestyle influences are also thought to be involved). In type three diabetes, the theory goes, the APOE4 gene somehow interferes with normal blood sugar uptake in the brain, thereby depriving the brain of the energy it needs to fuel cellular activities. Proof for it came in late 2000, when two psychiatrists – Eric Reiman at the University of Arizona, Tucson, and Gary Small at the University of California, Los Angeles – used brain imaging to show that people who have the APOE4 gene metabolise glucose at lower rates than people carrying the APOE2 or APOE3 versions.[8] Roses' followers don't have a nickname, but let's call them the 'E4ists'.

So, let's play out Roses' hypothesis. Over time, a brain starved of energy causes the functions of its neurons to decay, and like a city undergoing economic collapse, its service sector, or proteins, will start to malfunction – hence both the plaques and the tangles – until eventually the neuron gives up and self-destructs. But unlike other cell types, neurons can't replace themselves. So with each loss the energy burden on neighbouring neurons increases. And as an organ that constitutes 2 per cent of the body's weight yet requires 25 per cent of its energy, this is bad news for the brain. Unable to cope, more neurons self-destruct, a pathological cascade is initiated, and Alzheimer's takes hold.

For the goal of treating Alzheimer's effectively, both theories had their merits and pitfalls. Hardy's theory drew a straight line between amyloid and the disease, offering pharmaceutical tycoons an easy target. But it also imposed a narrative that was arguably too simplistic. And as 'seductive as this narrative might be,' one critic recently wrote, 'the dementing illness that we recognise as Alzheimer's disease is associated with a complex biology and biochemistry, as well as a pattern of brain disintegration that cannot easily be explained by a simple linear disease model.'[9]

Holding APOE4 responsible, on the other hand, would help plumb the genetic depths of old-age dementia, and perhaps help explain why amyloid formed plaques in the first place. But a gene that merely increased the chances of disease left drug discovery empty-handed. As one pharmaceutical magnate told me, 'Yes, APOE4 is by far the most prominent genetic link. But it doesn't *mean* anything. You can't offer someone who is APOE4-positive any therapy.'[10]

But there's a third option: what if neither theory could explain the disorder?

The fundamental precept of good science is that there is no place for beliefs. It's why scientists are repeatedly taught to replace 'believe' with 'think'. Enter our third group: the Tauists.

Tau stands for 'tubulin-associated unit'. It's the name of the protein that forms Alzheimer's tangles, the twisted knots of debris that seem to strangle neurons from within (the 'paired helical filaments' that Kidd and Terry spent years arguing about). Discovered in 1986 by three separate groups of researchers, tau normally acts as a kind of sealant for ropelike structures called microtubules, which stretch out along axons to create an internal transport system for every neuron. Scientists discovered that tau becomes tangled when it mixes with too much phosphorus inside the neuron. This tangled, hyperphosphorylated tau causes microtubules to fall apart. And that fact led the Tauists to assert their own hypothesis on the cause of Alzheimer's, which has come to be called, fittingly, the tau hypothesis.

Picture a zip-line whizzing sacks of crops between high-altitude villages in the tropics (farmers actually do this in Bolivia and other parts of South America). If the line comes apart, the crops won't reach their destination. For the neuron, those crops are neurotransmitters and biochemical nutrients, whizzing along the axon en route to synapses and other neurons. The failed deliveries have lethal consequences. Millions of synapses, the wellsprings of memory, will collapse and vanish. Then the axon itself begins to deteriorate, dying back until nothing but a limbless cell body remains. With all lines of transport and communication effectively terminated, internal chaos ensues and cell death becomes inevitable. When the neuron finally dies, all that's left are eerie coils of tau – what neuropathologists call 'ghost tangles'.

For Tauists, then, Hardy and Roses are both wrong. What's more, they have misunderstood the nature of Alzheimer's. There is no 'primary event' in the disease. Amyloid and APOE4 are just two triggers and there are probably many more. The crucial point was this: whatever triggered the disease, it all converged on a common end point – tau. It represented the 'how' behind neuronal death, when all else only represented the 'why'. It was, in short, all that truly mattered.

The idea had hefty support. Alois Alzheimer himself would have been more Tauist than Baptist. In 1911 he wrote: 'We have to conclude that the plaques are not the cause of [old-age] dementia but only an accompanying feature.'[11] And by the mid-1990s it had emerged that there are more than twenty brain diseases caused solely by tau malfunction – known collectively as tauopathies. If that wasn't enough to give tau the respect it deserved, argued the Tauists, nothing was.

At scientific conferences at the time the debate was raging. But the Baptists stood their ground. 'Tangles aren't particularly important,' Hardy told the *New York Times*'s Gina Kolata in 1995. He remains convinced that tangles are merely the result of plaques and therefore less worthy of our attention. It is inescapable that we should wonder how all this infighting actually helped patients. But such quarrels were and still are compulsory, because there are many theoretical paths for developing an effective drug. If we ceased thrashing out the best possible path, then the solution might take even longer to arrive.

I myself lean towards the amyloid cascade hypothesis, for the simple reason that amyloid appears to be where Alzheimer's begins. But I also think it unwise to assume that this fact somehow diminishes the relevance of APOE4 and tau tangles, because our understanding of causation remains unsophisticated. We still don't know, for instance, whether biological causes produce their effects by guaranteeing them: the inescapable fact that many people develop plaques yet remain cognitively healthy exemplifies that point. Thus, the cause of Alzheimer's is unlikely to be one single thing.

The most conspicuous flaw in the Tauists' argument was a lack of genetic evidence. Unlike amyloid, no mutations in tau were found in Alzheimer's patients, and without genetics as a guiding light, the idea of building a case against tau was like telling detectives to find a murderer by asking random people on the street. It was a messy lead, in other words. And at the start of a new century, the Baptists kept the upper hand, while the Tauists fast became renegades.

Meanwhile, steadily ticking over in the background, the world's largest, most ambitious biology project was under way: the Human Genome Project. Initiated in 1990 by the US Congress, the goal was to map every gene that made up a human being. Costing $3 billion and involving scientists in some twenty different countries, it was the biggest collaboration of biologists the world has ever seen.

On 14 April 2003, when the final draft was unveiled, it was heralded as the most valuable information humanity has ever known: 'More significant than splitting the atom or going to the moon,' declared Francis Collins, the project's US lead scientist; 'The most wondrous map ever produced by human kind,' announced US President Bill Clinton; 'The foundation of biology for decades, centuries or millennia to come,' said the UK lead John Sulston, who was to win a Nobel Prize for his work.

For Alzheimer's research it was game-changing. As the technology improved, thousands of patients rallied to have their genome sequenced, giving rise to genome-wide association studies (GWAS), in which small, previously hidden genetic variants could be uncovered. To date, more than twenty genetic variants have been identified – and the list will grow.

7

The Second Brain

Man is not made for defeat.
Ernest Hemingway, *The Old Man and The Sea*

THEY HAVE BEEN called many things – 'spider cells', 'little bags of poison', the 'other brain'[1] – but they are officially known as glia. Alois Alzheimer himself knew about glia; under the microscope they looked like scars bordering plaques and dead neurons. But like other scientists of his generation, he considered them little more than structural filler, and so for nearly a century they were overlooked. About thirty years ago, however, when scientists realised that glia constitute over half the human brain, they decided to take a closer look.

There are three types of glia.

Astrocytes: Greek for 'star cells' due to their shape, astrocytes are the largest, most numerous type. They control brain functions by mediating how neurons 'talk' to one another. In the hippocampus, for example, a single astrocyte contacts up to 140,000 neuronal synapses. In *The Other Brain*, astrocyte expert Douglas Fields argues that this behaviour is more complex than neurotransmission, meaning that higher mental faculties like consciousness, thoughts and feelings may actually be governed by astrocytes. They divide and die like other cells, and can grow uncontrollably in the most lethal type of brain cancer – glioblastoma.

Oligodendrocytes: Greek for 'few branched cells', they are the cellular factories of myelin, a fatty substance that insulates neurons by wrapping around their axons like the plastic sheath of copper wire. Myelin is white, hence the term 'white matter' as opposed to 'grey matter', referring to neurons themselves. A human's need for oligodendrocytes is darkly illustrated by multiple sclerosis, the devastating and common neurological condition caused by the widespread destruction of myelin. Without myelin, nerve impulses are disrupted, leading to fatigue, muscle weakness, visual problems and cognitive dysfunction.

And then there's microglia, literally 'small glia', the third and most important type for our story; these are the brain's immune cells. Swarms of these comparatively tiny cells orbit neurons in a surveillance state, constantly scanning them for signs of distress using long, antennae-like projections. In this mode they're dubbed 'resting' microglia. Once a threat is found, however, they transform from guard to soldier-at-arms. These 'activated' microglia then unload a payload of toxic chemicals to rid the brain of unwelcome guests such as meningitis and malaria.

This is important because in the late 1980s post-mortems revealed that Alzheimer plaques were often completely surrounded by microglia.[2] At the time no one quite knew what to make of this. But by 2001 advances in neuroimaging had made it possible to see activated microglia in living brains. In healthy people, the images nearly always showed a dim glow of activity across the brain. In Alzheimer's patients, though, the brain was lit up like a Christmas tree.

At face value it looked like a classic immune response – as if the microglia were attacking the plaques in a bid to eliminate them from the brain. The idea that the immune system could be involved in this way had radical and conflicting implications. On the one hand it suggested the brain was trying to remedy the problem from within; that we had, in effect, an ally on the inside. From this came the idea that perhaps the microglia just needed a helping hand, and that by artificially ramping up their healing power, the brain's immune system could be harnessed to treat Alzheimer's.

But this rose-tinted outlook was counterbalanced by something far less optimistic. Mounting evidence from cell culture research showed that microglia also appeared to kill neurons if their activation wasn't controlled.[3] I've done this experiment myself: leave microglia in a dish with neurons and a low dose of immune stimulant – fragments of bacteria or dead cells, for instance – and they will eventually turn on their neuronal neighbours.[4] Through the microscope the neurons look like a satellite image of a city at night, with the lights getting dimmer as clusters of circular bodies slowly blot them out.

This fact was once the bane of my existence. For two years I tested whether an experimental drug could hold off the microglia and allow the neurons to flourish. Every morning, including weekends, I entered the university, slipped on a white lab coat and blue rubber gloves, doused myself in sterilising ethanol, and had a look at how my cells were doing. What came next was usually the sight of dead neurons, an abrupt expletive (the standard response of a young scientist) and a phone call to cancel whatever social obligation I had planned. Others continue to work on the drug, but it's still unclear why the microglia do this to the neurons – whether the response is deliberate or just collateral damage.

In any case, the evidence suggested that the internal chaos of plaques and tangles might cause microglia to become dangerously overactive. These sabotaging cells could then start a deadly, self-perpetuating cycle of toxic inflammation, besieging the brain and driving the disease into a downward spiral. If that was the case, scientists had to wonder: would powering down the immune system help Alzheimer's patients?

Both scenarios were theoretical, of course, and arguably too simplistic. Microglia might be both good *and* bad for the brain. The answer depended on several unknowns, such as what state they were in when the disease started, how long they had been activated, and the role of genetic and environmental influences. But there was, unfortunately, precedent for the darker alternative. And two other types of dementia exemplify that point.

The first is neuroAIDS. In 1983, one year after the US Center for Disease Control and Prevention established the term AIDS to describe the opportunistic infection affecting young homosexual males, it was noticed that some AIDS patients also developed nervous system abnormalities similar to those seen in Alzheimer's. After experiencing a severe decline in memory, concentration, attention and language, they would end up bedbound and incontinent, usually dying three to six months later. It was often the earliest and sometimes only indication of a patient suffering from HIV. By 1987 researchers introduced the term 'AIDS dementia complex' to highlight the virus's impact on cognition, but it is now most commonly referred to as simply neuroAIDS. Although the anti-retroviral therapies released in the 1990s did appear to ameliorate neuroAIDS symptoms for some patients, exactly what combination of drugs was best suited for the purpose remained unclear. Today it's estimated that 10–25 per cent of HIV-infected patients develop this kind of dementia.[5]

But from a purely scientific standpoint neuroAIDS provides a powerful lens for pinpointing what brain changes are perpetuating the symptoms of Alzheimer's. NeuroAIDS is a disease with a known primary cause – a virus – and this gives scientists an opportune place to anchor their thoughts, because viruses are fixed entities in space and time and abide within well-defined parameters. Exploring this, scientists soon learned that after entering the brain the first cell type the HIV virus infects is microglia; neurons are spared until much later in the disease. That suggests that microglia, not neurons, are the core perpetrators of the symptoms of dementia.

Another form of dementia that gives a clue is called Nasu-Hakola, named after the Japanese pathologist and Finnish physician who first reported it in the early 1970s. This condition remains puzzling to this day. A patient with Nasu-Hakola first experiences severe bone fractures, usually during adolescence, in their hands, feet and knees. This can persist despite bone transplantation. Bizarrely, the young patient then develops a slowly progressing dementia, involving memory loss, personality changes, indifference and apathy towards those around them, problems with speech, and disorientation. Again, strikingly similar to Alzheimer's. By the mid-1980s researchers spotted that most cases were either of Japanese or Finnish descent, suggesting a genetic cause. And by 2000 geneticists had zeroed in on two culprit DNA mutations in the genes DAP12 and TREM2, both of which code for receptors on – you guessed it – microglia.

Suddenly microglia were in the spotlight. Experiments focusing on what their normal functions were and how mutations affected them were devised. Comparisons between Nasu-Hakola microglia and microglia in Alzheimer's were drawn. Therapeutic strategies to rein in their suspected overzealous behaviour were discussed. Scientists still weren't sure if they were allies or saboteurs; many ominously called them the brain's Jekyll and Hyde.

So when Dale Schenk, at a new company in San Francisco called Athena Neurosciences, wanted to empower microglia for an immune-based therapy on Alzheimer's patients, it was, to say the least, a bold move.

'I just had a simple idea,' Schenk told me over the sound of stirring teaspoons and soft chatter. Scientists don't usually meet under golden chandeliers and marble columns, but I'd managed to catch fifty-eight-year-old Schenk at a biotechnology conference being held at New York's illustrious Waldorf Astoria Hotel. His 'simple idea' was one so innovative that many scientists admitted they would never have thought of it. A vaccine for Alzheimer's.

We normally associate the term 'vaccine' with viruses and bacteria. Outbreaks of bird flu, Ebola and now Zika saturate the press with stories about the race to invent vaccines. But in pure biological terms, vaccines are any kind of agent that stimulates an organism to develop immunity. They can be dead or weakened forms of the threat itself – like Jonas Salk's polio vaccine and GlaxoSmithKline's chickenpox vaccine – or antibodies: blood cell proteins that label pathogens for destruction.

Schenk's vaccine for Alzheimer's was called AN-1792, and it consisted of synthetic beta-amyloid. His aim was to trick the brain into thinking that the plaques themselves were the foreign invaders, and thus stimulate a potent immune response. 'I thought, if we vaccinate mice with beta-amyloid,' he said, adjusting his glasses, 'they're going to develop antibodies to beta-amyloid and have them circulating in their blood, right? And a small fraction of those antibodies are going to get into the brain. Over time, that should disrupt beta-amyloid and dissolve the plaques.' Schenk grew up in Pasadena, California. The son of a fire chief and newspaper columnist, he went into science because 'it just seemed like a good idea'. After his PhD he worked on heart disease for a company called California Biotech. Then, one day in the mid-1990s, tired and frankly bored of the heart, he got talking to a colleague working on John Hardy's amyloid hypothesis.

'So what does beta-amyloid actually do?' Schenk remembered asking him.

'Oh, I don't know,' said his colleague.

'What do you mean you don't know?' urged Schenk.

'No one knows what it does, they just think it might cause Alzheimer's.'

'Well that's stupid. All it does is stick together. How could it cause Alzheimer's?'

The conversation continued in this vein until Schenk, finally convinced by the hypothesis, decided to join his colleague at Athena Neurosciences, where Schenk has now worked for the past twenty-eight years.

Perched on the edge of the San Francisco Bay, flanked by the brown sun-scorched slopes of San Bruno Park and Sweeney Ridge, Athena was the slick new contender that everyone thought would outsmart Alzheimer's. It had some of the brightest minds in the field – including Dora Games, inventor of the Alzheimer's mouse that provided support for John Hardy's amyloid hypothesis. With the amyloid hypothesis as its foundation, the company made a list of all the therapies it wanted to test in the mice.

Schenk's idea was low on that list. '*Nobody* wanted to do it,' he said, laughing. 'We had a list of thirty-three therapies we wanted to try on the mice and it was listed as number thirty-two. I couldn't even get any animals to do the experiment.' One of his colleagues thought the idea was so absurd that he put it on a list of bad ideas, which he stuck in the lab for all to see. As further ridicule, he gave Schenk the 'broken clock' award – even a broken clock is right twice a day – to which Schenk would retort, 'Well, at least it's *exactly* right twice a day.'

But with patience and dogged persistence, Schenk's time finally came. Managing to obtain a group of mice left over from somebody else's work, he performed the immunisation, sacrificed the mice, and sent their brains off for analysis. Then he waited. And waited – his gamble was hardly considered urgent – until, months later, he got a phone call from Dora Games herself. 'You're not going to believe this,' she said. 'But we're—'

'Not seeing any plaques in the mice that are vaccinated, right?'

So how did it work? I've spent years culturing microglia and can honestly tell you that we really don't know. The more we learn about microglia, the more complex their character turns out to be. Nonetheless, microglia tactics are basically twofold. They can secrete chemicals that kill parasites by degrading the parasite's DNA, or physically engulf the intruder in a process called phagocytosis (Greek, 'to devour'). Of course, Athena's neuroscientists didn't care how the patient's microglia chose to eviscerate the plaques, so long as they did it safely and stopped Alzheimer's as a result.

This now started to feel like an achievable feat. Between 1997 and 2000 vaccinations in rabbits, guinea pigs and monkeys all supported Schenk's discovery.[6] The vaccination even appeared to improve animal cognition. With that, the pharmaceutical companies Élan and Wyeth began human trials.

Human trials, also known as clinical trials, are typically split into four phases. Phases one and two are all about safety. In phase one the drug is given to a small group of twenty to eighty people to determine a safe range of doses. If no adverse effects are spotted the drug advances to phase two, where hundreds of people are treated and tests are performed to see if it has any biological effect. Most drugs, unfortunately, do not make it past phase two.[7] For those that do, phases three and four represent the peak of the mountain. In phase three thousands of people are tested over the course of several years; side effects are monitored; and if the drug appears to have worked it's then marketed and approved by agencies such as the FDA or EMA (European Medicines Agency). Phase four is a kind of follow-up to see how the drug is faring in the general population, and if there are any long-term effects that weren't detected earlier.

In a small phase one clinical trial of just twenty-four patients, a single dose of Schenk's vaccine appeared to be safe. Multiple doses were then given to more than seventy patients. Again, no adverse effects. Confident it was safe and worth pursuing, Élan and Wyeth moved to phase two, where 300 patients received the vaccine.

Scientists the world over were on tenterhooks. This was the first real-world test of the amyloid cascade hypothesis.

It was a disaster. Seventeen patients developed a dangerous form of brain inflammation called encephalitis, causing confusion, fever, and, if left untreated, seizures, stroke and death. In January 2002 AN-1792 testing was immediately aborted. After all the early promise it was a severe blow. And a hard lesson.

Schenk was stunned. 'Because we didn't see anything in the animals . . .' he lamented to me in a quiet, solemn tone, 'but it may have come and gone without us being able to detect it.' Determined the tragedy wouldn't be in vain, scientists around the world began an extensive follow-up of every patient from the trial. The findings were a mixture of encouraging, disappointing and just plain weird: encouraging because the first post-mortem showed a brain almost entirely clear of plaques; disappointing because Sid Gilman – Élan's elected expert to chair the trial's safety-monitoring committee – reported that of the 300 patients only 59 actually mounted an immune response; and plain weird because some patients did show a flicker of improved memory, even though a subsequent MRI scan showed that their brains had actually *shrunk*. How could a shrinking brain be found alongside increased cognition? 'We still don't know,' said Schenk. 'We may never know.' Only one thing was unanimously agreed: to watch every vaccinated patient like a hawk.

Four years later it was revealed that 159 patients did eventually show some improvements in cognition. Schenk's idea was alive again, and so if scientists could overcome the side effects then the makings of an effective treatment were in sight. Fortunately someone had already stumbled across a possible solution. Shortly after the trial ended, a Swiss psychiatrist named Christopher Hock found that patients who had made antibodies to beta-amyloid did better on tests of language, attention, memory and self-care than those whose immune system had not made antibodies.[8] Switching tactics, Schenk devised an antibody-based vaccine: Bapineuzumab, or 'Bapi', was an antibody made in mice but artificially tweaked for humans. The genius of this strategy was that patients would not have to mount a full-blown immune response because the antibodies to the plaques would already be present. It was less aggressive, and thereby reduced the risk of encephalitis.

In 2006 clinical trials were under way and the only side effect was a little water in the brain – cerebral oedema, quickly remedied by lowering the dose. By December 2007 the drug made it to phase three and more than 2,000 patients spanning North America and Europe, aged fifty to eighty-five, were enrolled.

It was the largest, most audacious attempt to combat dementia. Alois Alzheimer could only describe what he saw, William Summers could only delay the symptoms of the disease, but now Dale Schenk might be able to prevent the disease from taking hold. As the trial got under way, US pharmaceutical giants Pfizer and Johnson & Johnson stepped in, investing hundreds of millions of dollars in Bapi – the silver bullet to end an epidemic.

But it too failed. In August 2012 the results were in and Bapi showed no therapeutic benefit in all phase three trials, its effect on memory no better than a placebo. With the financial cost of the failure staggeringly high, Johnson & Johnson and Pfizer swiftly halted development.

There was widespread doubt over the amyloid hypothesis. Even early, highly influential supporters like Zaven Khachaturian – director of the NIA and recruiter of amyloid mastermind George Glenner – began to express reservations. 'The amyloid hypothesis became such a strong scientific orthodoxy that it began to be accepted on the basis of faith rather than evidence,'[9] he told one reporter, adding, 'no one has stepped back to ask whether our basic premise about the disease is the correct one.'

Schenk had his own doubts, but there were three gaping holes in the trial's design. First, how did we know these patients really had Alzheimer's? Post-mortem was still the only way to know definitively; perhaps they had another kind of dementia. Second, there was still no way of rigorously separating early from mid-stage cases; perhaps that skewed the overall result. And third, John Hardy and many other Baptists all agreed that the dose was too low; risks aside, there could be no kid gloves in this fight.

'We couldn't figure out who had the disease. We couldn't separate mild from moderate. And we were limited to low doses,' said Schenk. Another drawback, he explained, was the trial's benchmark for success. Because the activities of daily living vary so much between people – some people might do crosswords all the time, for instance, while others read or sew instead – the FDA demanded that trial candidates score highly on two different sets of cognitive tests, instead of the usual one. This set the bar for a positive result very high. 'So the sad part is that this drug probably would've worked for some people.'

Schenk's criticisms were soon backed up when scientists re-examined the drug using a powerful new technology. Pioneered at the University of Pittsburgh, Pennsylvania, 'PiB' (or Pittsburgh compound B) was a radioactive dye that bound to beta-amyloid in living subjects. Combined with conventional brain scans, PiB could actually show the spread of amyloid in the brain.[10] It was also a strong diagnostic tool: APOE4 carriers were more likely to show a bright PiB signal, as were carriers of APP mutations. But to the amazement of those involved in the Bapi trials, 30 per cent of the recipients were PiB-*negative*. They didn't have Alzheimer's. They had been misdiagnosed.

And so the flaws of the trials, along with the ambiguous nature of the results, gave researchers enough reason to continue pursuing vaccine therapy. They're still working on it today.

It was at this point that I had to ask: what did Schenk think caused Alzheimer's? He paused and breathed a heavy sigh. 'I don't think there's a single cause. I think it's like heart disease, and having plaques and tangles is like saying you have clogged arteries. You can have clogged arteries without having heart disease. And even though everybody views me as a Baptist, it's just that amyloid's been the most treatable drug target. That's why we've all focused on it.'

I told him about my conversations with John Hardy and Allen Roses, and how Roses had seemed disgruntled that people weren't paying enough attention to his APOE4 discovery. Schenk gave me a knowing smile. 'Well, John Hardy's a geneticist. Allen Roses is a philosopher. If he's disgruntled it's probably because he feels it's a target that we've missed, and he's probably right. But I swear to God we all tried our hardest to figure it out. Everybody had an APOE4 programme. We had one for eight years. Nothing came of it. That doesn't mean that APOE4 and the tangles are bad targets. It's just been harder to make a drug for them.'

Given all that, what will the cure look like? I asked. 'To be honest, I like to talk about *conquering* Alzheimer's rather than curing it. Because it's like asking, how do you cure heart failure? Well, you get a new heart. You can't get a new brain. So I think there's going to be a way to prevent it, or push it off many years. That's how we'll conquer it.'

I wasn't sure how I felt about his answer. Like many families and patients, I can't help but hope for something that reverses the symptoms altogether, rather than just holding back the disease –

something that reaches beyond the gloomy sea of dead neurons and pulls a memory back into the light. This might not be a fantasy (as we shall see in chapters fourteen and fifteen), but it's certainly further away.

One might wonder at the significance of these drug trials. With failures in the past the vaccine therapies have a lot to prove. I am yet to be convinced that a vaccine will work for everyone; Alzheimer's seems too nuanced for that. But if there's anything to provide real hope, it's a scientific lesson best articulated by a woman who was neither a scientist nor a physician. Gertrude Stein said: 'A real failure does not need an excuse. It is an end in itself.'[11]

We have known for a long time that the pantheon of science is decorated with failure. Failures are the moving force in science: they seal off one possibility in order to expose another; they force us to look at the problem in a new light. We owe a huge debt, therefore, to the researchers whose life's work leads to a cul-de-sac. They are indirectly showing us the correct path.

Altogether, these so-called 'prevention trials' promised a sea change in the fight against Alzheimer's. But while the concept of Alzheimer's as a process got scientists thinking about early prevention, this, they realised, depended critically and inexorably on something else: early detection.

8

Swedish Brain Power

Before we go any further, I just want to make it clear that I
don't want you to tell me that I've got Alzheimer's.

Anonymous patient's request to physician,
British Medical Journal, March 2014

THE MÖLNDAL HOSPITAL in Gothenburg, on the west coast
of Sweden, inhabits a complex of tall red-brick buildings
overlooking a wide expanse of countryside and wooden
houses. A highway cuts through this landscape, where a few taxis
huddle on a cramped collection point. Apart from the modern,
sky-blue trams gliding commuters to and from the city, it's a decidedly unremarkable place.

But within these ordinary walls, an intense and momentous
search is happening. The process uses drops of liquid so small, that
state-of-the-art robotics have been built specifically for the task.
They're looking for something Alzheimer's researchers have spent
the past two decades searching for: biomarkers – biological clues
observable long before symptoms appear, such as chemicals found
in blood and other bodily fluids. Anything, in other words, silently
lurking under the skin presaging a dark neurological future. After
the failure of Big Pharma's antibody trials, identifying biomarkers
for early intervention became the field's new priority.

The idea was far from new. In the mid-1990s scientists noticed
that beta-amyloid and tau also appear in spinal fluid, the colour-
less liquid enveloping the brain and spinal cord, providing

protective buoyancy as well as a good filtration system.[1] And, unsurprisingly, the levels differed between healthy people and those with Alzheimer's: beta-amyloid is reduced in the spinal fluid of Alzheimer's patients while tau is increased. Why they behave this way in spinal fluid isn't entirely clear, but we think it's because beta-amyloid becomes trapped in plaques inside the brain, while tau oozes out of the brain as neurons slowly fall apart. It has been found that this can actually happen twenty to thirty years before symptom onset. By the late 2000s, studies even showed that such observations could predict Alzheimer's with 90 per cent accuracy. A new 'pre-clinical' phase of Alzheimer's was coined in 2011, and scientists scrambled to find biomarkers wherever they could.

On a Monday afternoon in December 2015 I walked into the Mölndal Hospital and was greeted by a convivial man with a blond ponytail and a profusion of infectious energy named Henrik Zetterberg. In the wake of everything I'd learned about the expanding graveyard of drug tests, I'd travelled to Sweden hoping to glimpse a brighter, smarter future for clinical trials.

Growing up in the rural suburbs of west Gothenburg, near the stony reefs of the Kattegat Bay, Zetterberg spent his school holidays working in local nursing homes for extra pocket money. There, he saw first-hand the devastating effects of Alzheimer's, long before his classmates had even heard its name. His parents were not particularly academic, but when they spotted the young Swede's predilection for science, they encouraged him. His father started switching the radio on to listen to programmes by the Swedish molecular biologist Georg Klein, and Zetterberg became entranced by the intense, beguiling way he described a scientific conundrum. He went on to study medicine and, when it was time to specialise, probing the organs most accessible to physicians wasn't sufficiently Kleinesque for Zetterberg; he wanted to probe something that didn't surrender its secrets so readily. He specialised in clinical neurochemistry, and like an oceanographer studying the lakes and rivulets of the earth, Zetterberg set out to explore the hydrology and marine life of the nervous system.

Taking a seat in his office, I cut straight to the chase by asking how infallible these spinal fluid signals really were.

'We've been able to show that almost *all* people with biomarkers for plaques and tangles eventually develop Alzheimer's,' he told me in an astonished, surreptitious whisper. 'It's been one of the biggest, most important results in recent years.'

I was awestruck. In the future perhaps everyone would want to be tested. Perhaps the entire world would face the same choice as Carol and John Jennings.

With such a long time lag between disease initiation and mental collapse, Zetterberg thinks of Alzheimer's not as a thief in the night but rather a *Shawshank Redemption*-style escape artist. He thinks plaques and tangles are initially seeded in the brain during middle age – and then, like Andy Dufresne in his prison cell, they quietly start burrowing their way out. 'I think you start to get small seeds in your brain when you're forty or fifty – it's probably happening to me right now! – and that build-up lasts for decades. But it's not toxic, and beta-amyloid is basically sealed within plaques. But then something happens, and for about five to ten years you get new sub-seeds spreading. Then tangles form, the symptoms finally come, and the brain and hippocampus start to shrink.'

Zetterberg is certainly not shy of thinking outside the box. To see just how indicative of brain damage fluid signals are, he recruited the help of ice hockey players from the Swedish Hockey League.[2] This national obsession constitutes 288 professional athletes spread over twelve teams, and each player is only too aware of the risk of concussion and/or traumatic brain injury. 'It's really troubling them, because the sport is not about knocking someone out; it's about scoring, and these players have seen their teammates severely concussed.'

During the 2012–13 season, thirty-five players suffered concussions; some were so bad they knocked the player unconscious. Just before the season began, Zetterberg took blood samples from the players of two teams. He then repeated this on players at various time points after injury and found that tau – the main ingredient of tangles – rose in the blood within one hour following a concussion. He could use the levels to predict how many days it would take for the player to be well enough to return to play: the higher the level of tau, the longer it took for the player to recover.

Although the relationship between sports-related impacts and Alzheimer's is still debated, it's well established that boxing and American football can lead to other neurodegenerative disorders, such as Parkinson's and a dementing syndrome called chronic traumatic encephalopathy, respectively. These hard-hitting sports often cause the head to rotate rapidly – which, for nerve cell axons, creates a kind of shear, twisting physical force: the kind that bridges must contend with during high winds. It's a serious problem, and today Zetterberg is working with England's Saracens Rugby Club to develop impact sensors that detect these forces and instantly alert the player to take a break. Even for those of us who don't play these sports, his message is to avoid head injuries at any cost. The repercussions last longer than we think.

I didn't anticipate how much the disease exerts its influence completely under the radar, in a hidden and nebulous incubation period that scientists are only now beginning to comprehend. My understanding of the illness that robbed my grandfather of his twilight years was morphing and expanding into something totally different. A look into Zetterberg's lab changed the picture even more.

As we walked down the hall we passed an enormous piece of modern art. It depicted bolts of liquid flowing from a brain into a test tube, painted in bright hues of blue and orange. Stepping into the lab, it was clear what captured the artist's imagination. The entire room was abuzz with the sound of electronics and mechanics, unrecognisable contraptions the size of vending machines skirted the walls, and streams of polychromatic fluids fizzed through vast networks of clear hollow tubes.

'So here we have two robots,' Zetterberg said, pointing out two robotic arms injecting liquid into tiny plastic wells. I remember doing this technique by hand as a researcher; it was trying, to say the least. A technician was standing nearby, supervising the robots' progress. She told me the robots get through 200 samples of spinal fluid a week, half of which flag up a positive signal for Alzheimer's – or rather, future Alzheimer's. Testing people now doesn't make a lot of sense. With no cure or proven lifestyle countermeasure, little good can come from telling people they have a high chance of a harrowing illness. But Zetterberg thinks this will change in the future. 'That's why I really feel like we are prepared for the event of therapies,' he explained. 'In the future, when we get effective treatments, people in their forties or fifties will want to know. They will go to their physician and say, "My father had Alzheimer's and I would not like to end up like that. Could you please tell me if I'm biomarker positive or negative for the disease, and give me the treatment if I'm positive." I really feel like this is a realistic future.'

Zetterberg then introduced me to Dzemila, a young technician charged with organising all the data the robots churn out. Every day she trawls through hundreds of results for anonymised patients all around the world. 'There's someone from Sydney,' she says, pointing at the list on her computer screen. 'Prague . . . Copenhagen . . . Wisconsin . . . I don't like this list. I get panicked.' For Dzemila, it's not the disease but rather the exploding number of cases that frightens her. A single person's biomarker test takes seventeen minutes, she told me. The reason it's only performed on suspected Alzheimer's cases is because it simply wouldn't be ethical (until a proven treatment is found), not to mention feasible, to test everyone. I wondered whether I'd want the test; Alzheimer's was, after all, in my family.

Leaving Dzemila to her onerous list, Zetterberg and I continued the tour. He showed me robots testing spinal fluid by the *femto*litre (that's one thousand million millionths, or quadrillionth, of a litre). He showed me machines the size of small cars searching for biomarkers – our brain's neurological message in a bottle, it seemed. He spoke quickly, using wonderfully bizarre terms like *secretomics* and *electrochemiluminescence.*

I was amazed that humans were capable of building something like this. These tortuous amalgamations of tissue and technology were practically cybernetic organisms, with crystal balls for hearts. Then Zetterberg showed me the most important part of the lab, the biomarker discovery section – a bank of tall black boxes, each pulsing neon blue and green lights. It looked more like an NSA data centre than a neuroscience lab. Here, Zetterberg's machines are delving even deeper, looking for molecular clues besides beta-amyloid and tau, in mediums beyond spinal fluid. The problem with spinal fluid, Zetterberg explained, is that it requires an often painful lumbar puncture; it's too invasive. Blood is the next obvious choice because it's easily accessed, thus patients can be tested and followed over several years. He's already demonstrated proof of concept with his ice hockey concussion study. Now, others are extending this to Alzheimer's.

In March 2014 a group at Georgetown University, Washington DC, led by a neurologist called Howard Federoff, showed that differences in the levels of ten kinds of blood fats could predict whether a person is destined for Alzheimer's.[3] The changes were identifiable three years before symptom onset and were also 90 per cent accurate. In November of the same year Dimitrios Kapogiannis, an NIH researcher, claimed that defects in a blood-borne insulin protein called IRS-1 could predict Alzheimer's ten years in advance.[4]

But there are pitfalls. The numbers of patients enrolled in these studies were small, usually in the hundreds. Biomarkers are also hard to detect when submerged in four litres of blood (compared to 150 millilitres of spinal fluid). And the signals kept vanishing because substances alien to blood are quickly cleared.

Scott Turner, another Georgetown neurologist, suggested a more left-field approach in late 2013. At a conference that year he announced that Alzheimer's might be detectable in the eye. Using

Alzheimer's mice he found that the retina – a light-sensitive layer of neurons at the back of the eye – was up to 49 per cent thinner than that of healthy animals.[5] This extraordinary finding made headlines and may make more if it's replicated in humans. As one investigator observed at the time, 'It would be great if we could simply look into someone's eyes to see if they had Alzheimer's, but unfortunately spotting the disease is a lot more complicated than that.'[6]

Still, it's a start, and a very necessary one at that. After all, biomarkers promise much more than early diagnosis: they can turn drug development on its head. Because Alzheimer's unfolds gradually, effective drugs might work subtly and over lengthy stretches of time, making it hard to verify their true potency. A biomarker that reflects small biochemical changes could therefore reveal how well the drug is doing along the way. Whatever the outcome of biomarker research, my time in Zetterberg's lab made one thing abundantly and inexorably clear: this is one of the most exciting avenues of Alzheimer's research today.

Before I left Gothenburg, Zetterberg had one last thing to show me. It was something close to his heart, something that took him back to his childhood. We took a taxi from the hospital and drove towards the outskirts of the city. The streetlights receded in the distance and the light grew thicker in the wintry fog. We were heading to a government-funded nursing home in a borough called Frölunda, where the Swedes are experimenting with a new way of caring for Alzheimer's patients. I shouldn't say patients, though; that word has no place here. Here, they are residents.

We pulled up outside a white, modern, three-storey building, not far from the botanical gardens and the Göta älv River. Inside, Marika Mattsson, a member of staff casually dressed in a white shirt and jeans, welcomed us. After shaking hands, I glanced around the foyer and noticed something rather odd: there wasn't a uniform in sight. In fact, the place looked more like someone's house than anything else. Ninety-six residents live here, half of whom have dementia, the majority caused by Alzheimer's. It's one of many facilities scattered across Sweden to deal with the country's ageing demographic.

The Swedish government has served its citizens' longevity well. In recent years, the country pledged 4.3 billion Swedish krona to improve healthcare for the elderly, and Sweden now has one of the highest life expectancies in the world. By 2035 it's estimated that one in four Swedes will be over the age of sixty-five, and a 2013 United Nations report ranked Sweden the best country in the world for quality of life among the elderly (the UK ranked thirteenth; Afghanistan was the worst).[7]

Wandering the halls with Mattsson, it's easy to see why. The rooms are furnished with the tenants' possessions. Scores of kitchens and living rooms ensure that each only has six people in it at a time. There's a bakery, an art studio, a gym, even a spa (with a sizeable jacuzzi). What a contrast, I thought, to the asylum where Alois Alzheimer worked.

But it's the home's ethos that really makes the difference. The job of the staff here, as Mattsson sees it, is to give the residents a surrogate for their actual home. 'The key word is tranquillity,' she explained. 'We use small groups because we want to make this feel like a real home. And that's exactly what it becomes for many tenants. Sometimes, because they don't remember, we actually replace their relatives – we become their father, their mother, their brother, their sister, their old friend from school.'

Strolling into one room, Mattsson introduced me to a group watching a black and white movie. Some looked reasonably engaged; they were asking a young man sitting beside them to explain the movie. Others, of course, did not. According to Mattsson, many think they still have jobs to go to, and often dress and pack each morning in order to continue the careers they once had.

Also present were two relatives who introduced themselves as Annika and Mona and immediately invited me for coffee. Annika's seventy-five-year-old mother, Marie, has lived here for the past year, her symptoms having advanced beyond what the family could manage at home. They noticed symptoms eight years ago; in those days they'd find her fridge filled with exactly the same food products (twenty pieces of cheese for example). Marie also appeared to be storing money and personal possessions in clothes hanging in her wardrobe. Such innocuous idiosyncrasies soon transformed into indisputable omens when she began asking for her long-deceased mother and father. 'They're dead! Don't you know!?' Annika would reply in exasperation.

During her diagnosis, Marie underwent spinal fluid analysis, contributing to the first generation of patients receiving biomarker testing for Alzheimer's. Originally from Finland, Marie had moved to Gothenburg in her twenties and worked in a bakery before marrying a Swedish steel worker and settling down to raise Annika and her two siblings. In their mid-sixties, when the children had grown up and left home, Marie and her husband moved into a small three-bedroom apartment, ready to enjoy grandchildren and indulge in their long-sacrificed pastimes.

For Marie, that pastime was painting. Through her working years, she always maintained that she would one day paint the flowers she saw in magazines, routinely cutting out the pages portraying her favourite specimens. But by the time she'd bought a canvas and fashioned a palette, her symptoms forbade her from brushing a single stroke.

'I'm so mad at her for never painting,' said Annika, pouring herself another coffee. Her voice was calm and tender but frequently took on a hard-edged quality, as if the years watching her mother fade had inured her to Alzheimer's. She wasn't sad any more; she was angry. 'Now she's got hundreds of magazine clippings and dozens of canvases, and she keeps saying, "Oh I want to paint, I want to paint."'

I wondered what Marie's paintings would look like. I remembered the paintings of William Utermohlen, the American artist who lived in London. In 1995, upon learning that he had Alzheimer's, Utermohlen began painting a series of self-portraits. For five years he painted his face, each picture blurrier and more abstract than the last. The result was a staggeringly expressive portrayal of his descent into dementia, and the paintings were widely exhibited. But ironically, the very act of painting may have slowed his descent. Painting stimulates the parietal lobe, a region involved in creativity and one that remains intact until quite late in the disease. In the 2014 documentary *I Remember Better When I Paint*, therapist Judy Holstein explains:

> We know that [patients] take in colour, form, shape . . . and it translates in an Alzheimer's person's brain to have some meaning. The creative arts are an avenue to tap into a non-verbal, emotional place in a person. When they're given paint, markers, any kind of media for art making, and their hands are involved, and their muscles are involved, things are tapped in them that are genuine and active and alive. So the creative arts bypass the limitations, and they simply go to the strengths.

'I've tried to paint with her,' Annika continued, 'but she can't do it. She can't do anything any more. She spends all her time packing, because she thinks she's going home.'

The aim in Sweden is to keep the elderly and infirm at home for as long as possible. Independence, family and familiarity are seen as the best – if only – ways to preserve the mind and slow cognitive decline. Those who stay at home receive government aid, like home-delivered cooked meals. Some of Sweden's municipalities even arrange for small teams of elderly people to meet and cook together. The downside to this approach, of course, is that by the time people like Marie enter nursing homes they are heavily entrenched in their symptoms. In the opinion of Mattsson, this is problematic because many tenants then take at least six months to settle in. 'Today they're coming to us much later. The average age is between eighty-five and ninety, closer to ninety. When they come here they're so ill, so far into their dementia. And in the final stages of dementia you can't bond with people the way you once could, so it's harder to integrate them.'

To help Marie adapt to her new life in the home – and not wanting to see his wife exit life in fear and confusion – her husband has moved in with her. She doesn't recognise him, despite being married for fifty-six years. 'When she talks about her mother, my father just looks at me and sighs,' said Annika. 'She likes to sing Pavarotti. She keeps saying she will marry him. I say he is dead and your husband is sitting right there – don't talk about Pavarotti.' We all laughed. There's undoubtedly a droll kind of humour to Alzheimer's. It's often the best way to cope.

Fortunately, Marie's mind has yet to erase the memory of her children. And there are other things to be hopeful about. As she ventures through what the American essayist Susan Sontag called 'the night side of life', 'the kingdom of the sick',[8] Annika's mother – whether she knows it or not – played a small part in helping to decrypt Alzheimer's with biomarkers, and belongs to a society that cares for its night-side citizens with the wisdom, dignity and respect they deserve.

For the first time in my journey I sensed victory. Everything I'd learned about Alzheimer's represented mere snapshots of a process that evolves over decades. Up to this point, time had remained dementia's most intractable and elusive quality. But time, the murky borderland between health and disease, was the key. It may be simultaneously Alzheimer's great strength and Alzheimer's Achilles heel. And in Zetterberg's quest to exploit it, he was using it against Alzheimer's. He was doing what Shakespeare prescribed in *King John*:

> Be stirring as the time; be fire with fire;
> Threaten the threatener and outface the brow
> Of bragging horror.

He was turning the disease in on itself.

When we dream of a cure for Alzheimer's, we usually envision a pill for when symptoms appear. We forget that as our understanding of the disease is increasingly defined and adjusted, so too must our methods for defeating it be redefined, readjusted. It seems the bottom line in the world of drugs, science and medicine is that we need to spot the disease earlier. But what about the ordinary world? Are there lifestyle measures we can harness as well? Can we, in short, push it back ourselves in our daily lives? I wanted an answer.

PART III

Prevention

MY GRANDFATHER WAS not one for self-gratification. In the Islamic Republic of Iran he couldn't drink even if he'd wanted to. My father told me that he 'probably had six whiskies in his entire life, one for each time he visited us in England'. He kept fit, waking every morning at 5 a.m. to go hiking in the foothills of the Alborz Mountains in northern Tehran. He didn't smoke. And he had a good diet, eating plenty of fish, pomegranates, pistachio nuts and the vegetable-infused, rosewater-scented stews typical of Persian cuisine.

He lived a predominantly stress-free life too. A property developer in the affluent province of Shemiran, Abbas had inherited a fortune from his own father, Shaban, a logger and well-known figure in Tehran. Abbas was therefore free of financial worries, and in truth didn't need to work.

All told, my grandfather's decidedly salubrious life sheds little light on the cause of his illness. And this, I was beginning to realise, was a recurring theme: Arnold, the cultivated and bookish South African I met in London, lived a healthy life, as had Carol, the upbeat and proactive early-onset patient from Coventry. So what – if anything – destined a person towards dementia? More and more it was looking like the Californian neuroscientist Arthur Toga was right when he replied simply 'bad luck', in response to the same question posed by Terry Pratchett in 2008. Sardonically, Toga went on to say that 'this is an equal opportunity disease'.

But as I read the studies on lifestyle countermeasures – and there are many – it became clear to me that there is still cause for hope.

Though much of the evidence is preliminary and inconclusive, and sometimes merely anecdotal, considerations for stress, diet, exercise, cognitive training and even sleep are gaining scientific ground. And so I stepped into the uncertain world of preventive healthcare with cautious optimism.

9

Stress

There is more to life than increasing its speed.
Mahatma Gandhi, attributed

I N HIS TRAILBLAZING work *The Stress of Life*, published in 1956, endocrinologist Hans Selye explained how stressful experiences can make us sick. Before Selye, the notion that stress could influence our biology was practically unheard of. Today, we're all too familiar with the toll modern-life stress exerts on our health. Depression and anxiety, headaches, insomnia, heart disease: the evidence linking them to stress is overwhelming. Whether stress also contributes to Alzheimer's isn't as clear-cut, but once scattered and now mounting reports are giving weight to the idea.

Superficially it makes sense. The brain is the main organ controlling how we cope with stressful experiences, and all stresses lead to some kind of change in neuronal circuitry. In the short term these changes are good: they promote resilience, personal growth and learning. In the long term, however, when a person is repeatedly exposed to stress, they lead to neuronal wear and tear. And I mean that literally: animal studies show that repeated stress exposure shrinks neuronal dendrites, strips synapses, and even stunts the brain's ability to grow new neurons.[1]

Human brain imaging mirrors this sorry state. People with low social standing – that is, how a person ranks themselves within society – who report chronic stress have less grey matter in their prefrontal cortex.[2] There's even a report suggesting that three years after the 9/11 terrorist attacks, people who lived closer to the disaster had less grey matter in their hippocampus – the part of the brain that controls memory.[3]

Of course, the dimensions of human life are complex and multifarious. And the behavioural responses often associated with stress – diet, smoking, drinking, et cetera – make for a tangled web of cause and effect. That said, the evidence connecting stress to Alzheimer's is growing, not fading. Indeed, veterans who suffer post-traumatic stress disorder (PTSD) are nearly twice as likely to succumb to dementia, mostly as a result of Alzheimer's.[4] And Alzheimer's patients with higher levels of the stress hormone cortisol actually deteriorate faster.[5]

In the early 2000s a neuropsychologist named Robert S. Wilson at the Rush Alzheimer's Disease Center in Chicago devised a study to explore the link further. Wilson interviewed over 6,000 elderly volunteers from south Chicago using what psychologists call the 'neuroticism scale', a test where people are asked to rate their level of agreement on a five-point scale: 'strongly disagree', 'disagree', 'neutral', 'agree', 'strongly agree'. He then asked them to score a series of statements related to stress, such as, 'I am not a worrier', 'I often feel tense and jittery', 'I often get angry at the way people treat me', 'I often feel helpless and want someone else to solve my problems'. At the same time, Wilson assessed the participants using a battery of cognitive and memory tests.

Three years later he repeated the test on the same volunteers (bar the small proportion who had died), and three years after that began fishing for statistical evidence linking stress proneness to Alzheimer's risk.

The connection checked out. Of the 170 people who eventually developed Alzheimer's, the vast majority scored highest on the neuroticism scale. The data suggested that a stress–prone person is 2.4 times more at risk.[6] This finding was significant even after accounting for age, sex, race, education, medical history and posses-sion of the APOE4 gene. When Wilson carried out another similar study a few years later, the result was the same, only the odds rose to 2.7 times higher risk.[7] But how stress increases the risk of Alzheimer's remains a mystery.

In an attempt to demystify the link, researchers at the University of California, Irvine, led by behaviour expert Frank LaFerla, took mice and concocted a method to stress them out in a human, 'lifelike' way. LaFerla argued that early attempts to understand stress in Alzheimer's had failed because they'd looked at its effect over short time periods – minutes – or extremely long periods – days and weeks. This doesn't really reflect the reality of stress for humans, he said. So his team sought to 'mimic a short-term modern-life stressful experience, such as in car accidents and shooting events, which often last for hours rather than minutes or days/weeks'.[8]

LaFerla also pointed out that stress doesn't just arise psychologically; it's the result of physical trauma as well. He therefore wanted to stress the mice mentally and physically simultaneously. To do this, the mice were confined to small spaces and put on fast-moving platforms, all the while exposed to loud noise in a brightly lit room for five hours. Though these kinds of experiments do not sit well with me ethically, they have proved to be somewhat informative.

LaFerla's researchers then looked in the animals' brains. As expected, the mice's dendrites and synapses had shrunk compared to non-stressed mice. Unexpectedly, however, the stress also raised beta-amyloid levels and caused severe memory impairments that lasted up to eight hours. Translating those findings to the human world, LaFerla's team suggested that day-to-day stressful experiences – especially ones lasting several hours or more – might somehow accelerate Alzheimer's or at the very least worsen the disease in its early stages.

Over half a century ago Hans Selye wrote:

> Such expressions as, 'This work gives me a headache' or 'drives me crazy', grow out of experience . . . but there are *imperceptible tran-sitions* [italics mine] between the healthy, the slightly disturbed, and the insane personality . . . it is often the stress of adjustments to life under difficult circumstances that causes a change from healthy to disturbed, or from disturbed to insane.[9]

No doubt his choice of words is outdated. But the idea, for mental health and now Alzheimer's, perhaps resonates today more than ever: in our ceaseless endeavour to do and be more, we unconsciously integrate stress into the fabric of our everyday lives; we grant it acceptance and allow it to accrue; we forget that there are events in life where stress really is unavoidable (losing a job, getting a divorce, the death of a spouse). It's critical, therefore, to recognise when stress is avoidable and do our best to control it – because Alzheimer's is born of imperceptible transitions.

10

Diet

Let medicine be thy food and food be thy medicine.

Hippocrates

THAT PHRASE, WIDELY attributed to Hippocrates, has conjured up a host of novel nutrition fads, from the low-carbohydrate Atkins diet to the 'caveman' Palaeolithic diet, spawning an industry worth billions. They're so popular, in fact, that the evidence for many of these diets has taken a back-seat. We all know we should eat more fruit and fewer fats, more vitamins and less salt, but linking fixed diets to particular diseases is rocky terrain. Once again the problem lies in trying to prove causation based on observational studies. Nevertheless, there does appear to be some kind of relationship between Alzheimer's and diet.

In early 2015 a group of researchers in Chicago, led by a neurologist named Neelum Aggarwal, published a report suggesting that a Mediterranean diet might prevent Alzheimer's.[1] Aggarwal and her team observed the diets of nearly 1,000 people aged between fifty-eight and ninety-eight over four and a half years. They found that those who followed a hybrid diet, i.e. a Mediterranean diet combined with one that lowers blood pressure, were 52 per cent less likely to develop Alzheimer's. This included plentiful leafy vegetables, whole grains, fish, nuts and berries; minimal red meat, cheese, fried food, sweets and pastries.

Again, this is only an observation, but the link remained after factoring in the usual suspects: age, medical history, body mass index, education, depression and possession of the APOE4 gene. Moreover, a systematic review carried out at the prestigious Mayo Clinic in Minnesota concluded that 'while the overall number of studies is small, pooled results suggest that a higher adherence to the MeDi [Mediterranean diet] is associated with a reduced risk of developing MCI [mild cognitive impairment] and AD [Alzheimer's disease], and a reduced risk of progressing from MCI to AD'.[2]

How does what we eat protect us? It's all due to a foggy connection between the brain and the gut. Collectively known as the microbiome, the bacteria that reside symbiotically inside us are vital to brain health. This was demonstrated most starkly in November 2014, when Swedish researchers at the Karolinska Institute in Stockholm showed that germ-free mice – gnotobiotic mice, housed and fed inside sterile containers – are born with leaky, defective blood–brain barriers.[3] The blood–brain barrier is a wall of cells that decides what can and cannot enter the brain from the blood coursing through its capillaries. In Alzheimer's, it's one of the first things to break down, especially around the hippocampus, where memories are made.

But the microbiome can be a dangerous bedfellow too. If excessive amounts of bacteria breach the blood–brain barrier, they will activate the brain's immune cells – microglia, the cellular protagonists of the Alzheimer's vaccination story in chapter seven – and cause a form of inflammation that weakens the blood–brain barrier even more, setting in motion a vicious cycle in which more bacteria are let in and more inflammation ensues.

An irresistible case for this very scenario happening in Alzheimer's was made six years ago by a Swiss-Hungarian neuropathologist named Judith Miklossy. She found that the density of bacteria is eight times higher in Alzheimer's brains than in healthy people.[4] Spirochaetes, the spiral-shaped variety of bacteria, were the main culprit. They have 'the ability to invade the brain, persist in the brain and cause dementia', Miklossy wrote. She also pointed out that dementia is a feature of late-stage Lyme disease, an infectious disease caused by the *Borrelia* bacterium. These micro-organisms can evade host defence mechanisms and ultimately help lead to the formation of plaques and tangles.

It turns out that the Mediterranean diet is filled with anti-bacterial foods – such as garlic, olive oil and honey. Cinnamon also weighs in, with one study demonstrating that cinnamon extracts fed to Alzheimer's mice shrink plaques and improve cognition.[5]

Since writing this, a randomised clinical trial – the gold standard for assessing interventions, where participants are randomly assigned to either a treatment or placebo group to reduce bias – has been done on the role of diet in age-related cognitive decline (that's not Alzheimer's, of course, but experts agree this may apply nonetheless). Sweden's Karolinska Institute was again leading the way. In what they dubbed the 'Finnish Geriatric Intervention Study to Prevent Cognitive Impairment and Disability,' or FINGER, scientists randomly assigned over 1,200 sixty- to seventy-seven-year-old Fins to a strict, two-year diet, and those who followed the diet did significantly better on cognitive tests than those who did not.[6]

As someone who obsesses over those colour-coded boxes divvying up food groups on food packaging, I loved the details of the study. The diet was as follows:

> 10–20% of daily energy from proteins, 25–35% daily energy from fat [less than 10% saturated fat, 10–20% mono-saturated fatty acids, 5–10% polyunsaturated fatty acids, and 2.5–3 grams per day of omega-3 fatty acids], 45–55% daily energy from carbohydrates [less than 10% from refined sugar], 25–35 grams per day of dietary fibre, less than 5 grams per day of salt, and less than 5% daily energy from alcohol.

In plain English: 'These goals were achieved by recommendation of high consumption of fruit and vegetables, consumption of wholegrain cereal products and low-fat milk and meat products, limiting of sucrose intake to less than 50 grams per day, use of vegetable margarine and rapeseed oil instead of butter, and fish consumption at least two portions per week.'

Reading the study, I was almost disappointed. This advice has been a common narrative among doctors and dieticians for years. Now, however, we may have even more cause to listen.

II

Exercise

It is exercise alone that supports the spirits, and keeps the mind in vigour.

Cicero

FOR MANY, THE top seed in the race for lifestyle interventions is exercise. This is somewhat surprising considering the lack of hard evidence. But there's an intuitive logic here that is somehow hard to dismiss. Suffice to say, the overall health benefits of physical activity are considerable. Even moderate exercise can markedly lower blood pressure and improve cardiovascular health. And it is these resulting rewards that are thought to directly affect Alzheimer's risk.

Having high blood pressure in middle age, for instance, puts one at higher risk of Alzheimer's.[1] Conversely, if one's blood pressure is too low, especially over the age of seventy-five, the chance of Alzheimer's still increases.[2] Why? That's unclear. Most evidence points towards a link between blood pressure and inflammation (again involving microglia), but exactly how this feeds into the whirlwind of plaques, tangles and brain calamity remains an enigma.

What is conclusive, in lab mice at least, is that exercise on a treadmill can reduce the build-up of plaques and tangles.[3] This modest miracle is thought to happen by activating an intriguing cellular phenomenon called autophagy (Greek for 'eating of self'), a specialised kind of cellular housekeeping that clears out damaged or unwanted goods and introduces new ones after recycling the old, all as part of an adaptive and protective process to help neurons better cope with stress and extend their lifespan. So it's thought that stimulating autophagy through exercise may halt the progression of brain cell death in Alzheimer's.

To take the molecular parlance a step further, a protein called BDNF (brain-derived neurotrophic factor) is the leading actor in this subplot. In December 2010 researchers at the University of Pittsburgh, Pennsylvania, recruited 120 people with an average age of sixty-seven and had them perform either moderate aerobic exercise or simple stretches three days a week. Strikingly, follow-up MRI scans revealed that those who exercised netted a 2 per cent increase in the size of their hippocampus.[4] That isn't bad considering that 1.5 per cent shrinkage is normal for this age. And the middleman in this small victory, it appeared, was BDNF: a molecule known to promote the birth of new neurons and synapses throughout the entire nervous system. BDNF has such potent effects on neurons, moreover, that pharmaceutical companies now view it as a good drug candidate, causing some scientists to whimsically grant it the rather droll nickname 'brain fertiliser'.

Such a wonder is, sad to say, perhaps decades away. So in the meantime we must resolve not only to exercise but also to learn what kind of exercise and how often it's required to keep the mind fit. The most thorough investigation of the subject so far – a systematic review entitled 'The effect of exercise interventions on cognitive outcome in Alzheimer's disease' by researchers at the University of Sussex, England, in 2014 – could find several methods demonstrating positive effects on cognition in Alzheimer's patients.[5] They ranged from thirty minutes of walking (four times a week for twenty-four weeks), to one hour of cycling (three times a week for fifteen weeks), to thirty minutes of vigorous calisthenics (every day for twelve weeks). For those who have reached an age where even walking is a chore, gentle movements, such as those practised in the Chinese martial art Tai chi, were also deemed worthwhile.

The fact that both high- and low-intensity exercise appears to help speaks volumes. Larger studies are still needed to unequivocally prove a link with Alzheimer's, and this certainly doesn't mean that someone can avoid the malady simply by working out. This brand of science – epidemiology – dispenses truths about millions, not individuals. Indeed, my grandfather's quotidian hike lasted two hours. But still, a little exercise is probably worth it.

Naji Tabet, chief author in the investigation and a lifestyle research front-runner, emphasised this point when I spoke with him on the telephone. 'You do not have to run marathons. You do not have to go to the gym three or four times a week. A brisk walk will do!' Tabet decided to focus on exercise as a way to prevent Alzheimer's out of desperation more than anything else. 'When you see an illness that robs someone of their personality, their individuality, an illness that ravages their life and the life of their loved ones, you have to treat it in whatever way you can.'

Tabet has looked at what fitness fanatics call Ultra Vets, people in their seventies or eighties who exercise religiously. (I've worked in a lab with someone who fits that description; he was eighty-two years old, had not retired, and had just trekked across the Antarctic.) When Tabet compared a group of Ultra Vets who had no memory problems with an age-matched group of people who do what you or I would say is a normal amount of exercise, he found *no difference* in cognitive skills between the groups. 'So if you overdo it,' he said, 'there's diminished returns. Just do low-intensity exercise. Keep the heart going, keep the muscles going, keep the respiratory system going. Even a couple of minutes a day might protect you.'

But still I wondered, how is this possible? 'Nobody knows exactly how it works,' Tabet granted. 'My feeling is that exercise helps the immune system fight the build-up of plaques and tangles. But exercise also helps the mood. And we know that people who are depressed are more at risk of Alzheimer's, so it might have an indirect effect by simply making somebody feel better.'

Fantastical though it might sound, Tabet also thinks that mild exercise can go a step further than prevention. He believes it may actually slow the decline of Alzheimer's in late-stage patients. He insists that activities as simple as throwing a ball around, gently moving the arms and legs, stretching – anything, in other words, that meets his explicit and unadorned message to 'keep things going' – will do something.

With that, remaining positive, I moved on to rediscover a different form of exercise altogether.

12

Brain Training

Anyone could be seduced by research when the results poured in. The trick was to love it when the results weren't forthcoming, and the reasons why were elusive.

Lisa Genova, *Still Alice*

IN 2001 FORTY-ONE-YEAR-OLD Japanese physician Ryuta Kawashima began investigating the effects of video games on the brain. Based at Tohoku University in Japan after conducting neuroscience research at the Karolinska in Sweden, he already knew that functional brain imaging was his vocation; he found the hypnotic quality of seeing thoughts flash across a screen irresistible: here was a living map of the mind that responded to the observer like reflections in a mirror. Two years later, he published a book containing quirky cartoons of people performing daily activities next to miniature pictures of brains lighting up in response. He included straightforward mental arithmetic and various puzzles and quizzes – all, as the book clearly states, 'to help you rejuvenate your brain and develop its functions to a higher level'. It was the author's dream to make brain health maintenance 'a social priority'. And in 2005 his dream manifested as a global sensation: the celebrated Nintendo *Brain Training* video game.

I've never been much good at Kawashima's famous game. I was somewhat surprised to hear it's been touted as a way to prevent Alzheimer's – I didn't think people took it seriously in health, let alone disease. But believe it or not, for over a decade it has been used in thousands of nursing homes across Japan in a desperate attempt to do precisely that.

A mere glance at some demographics explains why. The East Asian island nation is now home to the fastest ageing population on the planet. Nearly a third of its citizens are above the age of sixty-five, and this is set to climb to 40 per cent by 2055.[1] Combine that with the estimated drop in Japan's population from 127 million to 90 million in the same timespan – due to notoriously low birth rates – and it's not surprising that the country is on the brink of a dementia epidemic. The dire situation has led the Japanese minister of health to call for a million extra foreign nurses and carers by 2025, to thwart a population collapse.

So, does it work? Kawashima certainly thinks so. 'I believe that the brain is a brain, whether it's in children or older people.' Kawashima was sitting opposite me in his office at Tohoku University in the northern Japanese city of Sendai. I'd become too fascinated by the idea of a computer game treating Alzheimer's to miss the opportunity of a face-to-face meeting with him. 'I know that naturally the brain deteriorates during the course of ageing, but I think that we can maintain a certain level of cognitive function using *Brain Training*.'

'Even with Alzheimer's?' I asked.

'Sure!' Kawashima replied, almost surprised by the question. He told me that more than 30,000 people are using *Brain Training*, and that the effect in nursing homes is dramatic. 'People frequently ask me to visit their nursing home, in fact. They say they are seeing unbelievable changes. I didn't believe it at first; I thought, they tell me a lie. But then I went and it was true. Patients who were doing nothing before, just sleeping and sitting in a wheelchair, were doing simple arithmetic problems.'

I couldn't help but be struck by Kawashima himself. He was immaculately dressed in a long black suit and looked twenty years younger than his fifty-six years of age. He has a calm, gentle manner, which I soon realised betrayed a supreme underlying confidence. Despite the scepticism surrounding his invention – not to mention being branded a charlatan by some of his peers – he seemed somehow above it all. He wasn't trying to cure Alzheimer's. He was simply trying something new and wildly innovative; something that just might buy patients a little extra time.

Perhaps the most striking observation, though, was the fact that his bookshelves were filled in equal measure with books and Nintendo DS games. He pulled one down to show me. 'This is Nintendo *Concentration Training*. It is very hard. In Japan it's called devilish training.' He pointed to a picture on the cover. It was a picture of the familiar animated floating head of Kawashima. 'Look, here is my face as a devil!' he exclaimed, laughing.

'This is too hard for people with dementia, of course, but now I am interested in the prevention of dementia. And as you know, the beta-amyloid and tau proteins are already accumulating in the brain from age forty to fifty, so I believe we must all do brain training regularly before age forty.'

Before meeting Kawashima, I'd done some digging into the scientific veracity of cognitive training. Some researchers believe that any positive effects are due to something called the Hawthorne, or observer, effect, in which people change their behaviour when they know they're being observed, internally vocalising particular tasks, for instance, that might improve their score but don't reflect any underlying improvement in cognition. Others argue that the brain remains modifiable throughout life, and that we simply haven't developed the right tools to see how everyday experiences can affect it.

In September 2009 the Alzheimer's Society funded a huge trial involving more than 13,000 people. They found that while cognitive training did nothing for people under the age of fifty, it did help those over sixty with everyday tasks such as shopping, memorising lists and overseeing finances – provided they play it for ten minutes, five times a week for six months.[2] Improvements like these can last for up to five years, some researchers say. In more visceral terms, cognitive training has actually been shown to improve blood flow to the prefrontal cortex – a region so integral to human thought it's been called the 'organ of civilisation' – and strengthen nerve connections between brain hemispheres in seventy-year-olds.[3]

On whether it's an Alzheimer's deterrent, the simple answer is: we still don't know. A few reports suggest it might work. In 2012, for instance, a US group spent five years investigating 700 people over sixty-five and found that those who frequently did crosswords and puzzles, or played cards and checkers, were 47 per cent less likely to develop Alzheimer's.[4] But the study was bedevilled by its modest size, leaving many unconvinced.

Consider this by cognitive neuropsychologist André Aleman, who wrote in 2014: 'Cognitive training is nothing more than practising mental capacities such as memory, concentration, and thinking skills . . . [and] is often extremely specific, while the decline is across the board. So if you do a lot of Sudoko puzzles, you become extremely good at Sudoko puzzles, but your brain hasn't necessarily become sharper in other areas.'[5]

But while emphasising that the research behind *Brain Training* is still in its early days, Kawashima left the door open to the immensely powerful effect he believes the game has on the brain. 'We know that the prefrontal cortex is activated by brain training,' he said, 'and the prefrontal cortex plays many roles in higher cognitive functions – like memory, attention and decision-making. So if we can stimulate the prefrontal cortex in one way, then basic functions of the prefrontal cortex must improve. That's my hypothesis.'

It sounded reasonable enough to me – certainly enough to make me want to pick up my old console and devote some time to it before I turn forty. Here in Japan, the Mecca of the video-gaming world, I realised that this game is not just an entertaining gimmick: it's a purposeful and evolving technology. Indeed, Kawashima is trying to dissect its neurological effects using an experiment he calls neurofeedback, wherein a person can see their brain activity on a computer screen while playing the game, and has to concentrate on trying to control certain patterns of activity by focusing more or less on different aspects of the game. Unsurprisingly, Nintendo continue to watch Kawashima's research closely.

Kawashima is certainly no snake oil salesman, though. He turned down a €15 million pay cheque for his invention, and still refuses to keep any of the $30 million amassed in royalties.

'My wife is not happy with that,' he told me, grinning.

'Why didn't you keep any of it?' I asked in disbelief.

He shrugged. 'I didn't feel it belonged to me. I just did my job as staff at the university. And my salary is paid for in taxes by the Japanese people, so I felt it belonged to the university.'

Kawashima has channelled the game's profits into research at Japan's Tohoku University, where he now leads a group of forty young neuroscientists. Two of them – Susumu and Akira – offered to show me around the lab. In a starched white room inside a building opposite Kawashima's office, they were testing *Brain Training* on mice. Well, not quite. But the experiment they've set up is a pretty neat simulation. First the mice live in bare, empty cages, with hardly anything to stimulate their brains. Then they're moved to an 'enriched' cage, containing toys, tunnels, multiple floors and a maze which Akira changes three times a week to outfox them. Using a specialised mini-MRI machine, Akira then has a look at their brains. 'I'm looking for signs of plasticity,' he told me, 'changes in the structure and connectivity of the brain.' Astonishingly, every time Akira trains his mice using the enriched environment, their brains get bigger. And here's the crucial point: this happens with both old mice *and* transgenic Alzheimer's mice.

Akira thinks it might have something to do with another relevant theory called brain reserve. Conceived by an American geriatric researcher named James Mortimer, the idea is that each person's brain holds a certain amount of resistance to mental decline, irrespective of how much structural damage has actually occurred. Mortimer believed brain reserve is intrinsically linked to the amount of mental stimulation a person engages in throughout life: the greater the stimulation, the greater the brain reserve. He was convinced it was the reason people could have plaques in their brains without ever experiencing dementia.

In 1990 Mortimer teamed up with epidemiologist David

Snowdon to study brain reserve in a group of highly educated centenarian nuns at the convent of the School Sisters of Notre Dame in Mankato, Minnesota. Snowdon believed nuns were perfect candidates for such a study. Their uniform living arrangements and exceedingly regular diet and exercise regimes helped rule out conflicting variables, allowing a more focused look at the role of education. The sisters' fastidious record-keeping also meant he had access to medical and historical records dating back to the late 1800s. Among these records were collections of autobiographical essays that the nuns had written as part of their inauguration to the convent, when they were in their early twenties. By analysing the essays' grammatical and linguistic sophistication – what Snowdon called 'idea density' – he discovered a strong connection with Alzheimer's.

For example, a sister describing her siblings was more likely to get Alzheimer's if her essay read like this: 'There are ten children in the family six boys and four girls. Two of the boys are dead.' As opposed to a sister whose essay read like this: 'Already two, a brother and a sister, had begun the family which would gradually reach the number of eight . . . When I was in the fourth grade death visited our family taking one to whom I was very particularly attached, my little brother, Karl, who was but a year and a half old.'

An incredible 90 per cent of the sisters with low idea density went on to develop Alzheimer's, and from these essays alone – essays written some sixty years earlier – Snowdon could predict with 80 per cent accuracy which sisters would do so.

The amazing findings of the 'Nun Study', as it became known, prompted a wave of media interest. One nun even appeared on the cover of *Time* magazine behind the catchline: BELIEVE IT OR NOT, THIS 91-YEAR-OLD NUN CAN HELP YOU BEAT ALZHEIMER'S. As Snowdon wrote in *Aging with Grace*:

> We now know that the brain is capable of changing and growing throughout life, but there is no question that most of its growth comes during our earliest years . . . Parents ask me if they should play Mozart to their babies, or buy them expensive teaching toys,

or prohibit television, or get them started early on the computer. I give them the same simple answer . . . 'Read to your children.' [6]

Brain reserve, if real, is a developmental phenomenon. But what it offers is lifelong neuroprotection.

For Kawashima, though, flexing the mind in adulthood is far from too late. And with Japan's booming Alzheimer's epidemic, his mission is now more urgent than ever. 'My future is to succeed with prevention,' he said as I bade him goodbye. 'That's my hope . . . My dream.'

13

Sleep

Sleep is a rose, as the Persians say.

Vladimir Nabokov, *Lolita*

NO ONE KNOWS why we sleep. The obvious answer is that we do it because we're tired. But the brain is 95 per cent as active during sleep as during our waking hours. And that, given our evolutionary legacy as prey for larger predators, not to mention the amount of time we lose for reproduction and food gathering, makes the reason for sleep all the more mysterious.

For decades there have been theories to better explain it, ranging from wound healing and heat regulation, to memory consolidation and dream-induced creative thinking. But recent work, published in leading scientific journals, suggests that sleep may also exist to shield the brain from Alzheimer's.

It began in 2005, when a group of psychiatrists at St James Hospital in Dublin demonstrated a link between sleep disturbances, like increased insomnia and daytime sleeping, and the severity of dementia in their Alzheimer's patients.[1] This didn't come as a surprise – many brain disorders correlate with sleep disturbances – and so it was mainly viewed as practical knowledge to help doctors and caregivers choose the right medicine to help their patients sleep.

But others believed the link was more far-reaching; that something deeper was at play. So scientists set about replicating the paradigm in Alzheimer's mice.

Among them was a group at Washington University, St Louis, led by a man named David Holtzman. His team showed that beta-amyloid levels fluctuate with sleep–wake cycles: depriving mice of sleep raises beta-amyloid levels, while chemically stimulating sleep lowers them.[2] That was 2009, and the discovery was soon supported by the group's converse observation, in 2012, that vaccinating the mice against beta-amyloid restored normal sleeping patterns.[3]

One year later, Maiken Nedergaard and her team at the University of Rochester, New York, found evidence that the brain actually cleans itself during sleep,[4] removing beta-amyloid using a network of microscopic channels filled with spinal fluid called the glymphatic pathway: a kind of plumbing system composed of glial cells that clears the brain of waste products. She compared the sleeping brain to a 'dishwasher' clearing out molecular 'dirt'. The findings were impressive. The only nagging caveat was that mice (besides being mice) are nocturnal; they have different sleeping behaviours to us. A human study was desperately needed.

This came from researchers at the University of California, Berkeley, led by a neuroscientist called Matthew Walker. For Walker, a young, fresh-faced, jocular professor originally from England, sleep is more intimately tied to memory than people realise. He likes to preface his lectures by assuring people that they are allowed to fall asleep during his talk. 'Knowing what I know about the relation-ship between sleep and memory,' he recently told one audience, 'it's actually the greatest form of flattery, for me, to see people like you not being able to resist the urge to strengthen what I'm telling you by falling asleep.'[5]

In July 2015 Walker and his team recruited twenty-six healthy people with an average age of seventy-five, and set out to uncover the relationship between sleep, beta-amyloid and memory.[6] To begin, Walker performed PiB-PET scans on the recruits to gauge their brain's amyloid quota. Then he made the participants memorise sets of word pairs before asking them to spend the night in a sleep laboratory, where their sleeping patterns could be professionally monitored.

Sleep moves in roughly ninety-minute cycles, made up of rapid eye movement (REM) and non-rapid eye movement (NREM) phases. REM sleep only lasts around ten minutes and happens while dreaming (though why the eyes move is unknown). Deep and dreamless NREM sleep dominates each cycle, but becomes less dominant later in the night as REM sleep encroaches slightly more into its time. Memory consolidation is thought to occur during an NREM phase called slow-wave sleep – a period of synchronised, low-frequency pulses of electrical activity. This is what Walker was particularly interested in for the human study.

The next morning, Walker's recruits retook the word-pair test during a functional MRI brain scan. As it turned out, the participants with the highest beta-amyloid levels had the lowest slow-wave activity and scored the worst on memory recall. The reduced slow-wave activity was most prominent in the prefrontal cortex – the brain region where beta-amyloid accumulation was at its highest. This was seen after correcting for age, sex and brain size. What's more, the participants were told to abstain from stimulants such as coffee and alcohol two days before testing. Mathematically, there is a linear relationship by which beta-amyloid affects sleep, which then affects memory. This makes sleep itself a possible candidate for therapeutic intervention in Alzheimer's. Walker published the study in *Nature Neuroscience* and, predictably, received full-bore sensationalism from the press.

But there are two problems with the study. First, the findings are correlative: they don't prove cause and effect. For that, people's sleeping habits would have to be followed over several years. Second, it's possible the results were swayed by the recruits' having to sleep in a new environment. Walker had asked them to make home sleep logs and told them they could sleep in the laboratory in the same way, but without somehow measuring the difference between the two settings, the findings remain open to interpretation.

Which is precisely what Holtzman and fellow neurologist Brendan Lucey have done. 'Despite these issues,' they wrote in an opinion article accompanying the study, 'the study by [Walker's team] provides important new insights into the changes in sleep and memory in preclinical Alzheimer's disease, as well as indicating potential new avenues for investigation.'[7] They've argued for alternative ways that the trifecta of beta-amyloid, sleep and memory are connected. According to them, it may be that beta-amyloid affects sleep and memory simultaneously, or that sleep problems associated with ageing affect memory and beta-amyloid, which in turn affects sleep, creating a self-perpetuating loop of havoc. How tangles fit into this is unknown. But hurdles aside, few would dispute the importance of a good night's sleep, and this blossoming new area of research wholly and irrefutably strengthens that mandate.

What are we to make of so much ambivalence? If my grandfather were alive today, he'd probably tell you to live like a rock star; the austere life he led certainly didn't protect him. But still, there's no denying that the evidence for non-pharmacological countermeasures against Alzheimer's, albeit conflicting, exists. Of course, as a scientist, I'd be the first to say that evidence alone isn't enough – it has to be *good* evidence: large samples, widely replicated, and so forth – but since we know that these lifestyle measures are good for us anyway, the most sensible approach is to play it safe. So follow a Mediterranean diet. Exercise. Avoid stress. Stimulate your mind. Sleep. You've got nothing to lose and everything to gain.

PART IV

Experimentation

IN OCTOBER 2012, shortly after Abbas passed away, I attended the Society for Neuroscience conference in New Orleans, Louisiana, with almost 30,000 fellow neuroscientists. The conference has been a pilgrimage for researchers since its founding in 1969. It's where the most dedicated academics gather to present data and share ideas. I had just finished the second year of my training and this was my first taste of international collaboration at the highest level. And it did not disappoint. For five glorious days I met and spoke with people conducting the most advanced experiments the world has ever seen. Each morning I was handed a hefty catalogue outlining the day's presentations – you have to plan your day meticulously if you're to see even a fraction of what's on offer – and each morning I immediately flipped to the section on Alzheimer's.

My first feeling, as I wandered the endless corridors of lecture theatres and poster exhibits, was a hypnotic mix of awe, intrigue and frustration. So numerous were the breakthroughs and new theories, I wanted to clone myself and put a copy of me in every room. I wondered if my research using the brain's immune cells was still cutting-edge. Like an octopus, the field appeared to have spread its arms into wholly uncharted territory.

One evening that week, alone in my hotel room, I received a Skype call from my father. Like others in my family he wanted to know if I'd spotted anything that might have helped Abbas. I told him that the research here was experimental and probably wouldn't have done much for Granddad. I could see the disappointment on his face. I think that after seeing Abbas's decline he had grown fearful of dying in the same way. In the year preceding his death, the most visible change in Abbas's personality was his inconsistency: snapshots from the past – a familiar piece of music, say, or an old photograph – prompted sudden sprees of mirth and coherence, while prolonged moments of introspection hurled his mind into a labyrinth of jittery, existential unknowns.

I think my father would have tried anything at that point, and a part of me felt as if I'd failed him. I still had nothing to offer even with an army of neuroscientists by my side. It's a reality every researcher confronts. Try as we might, there's an infuriating spectral quality to research on the front line: a promising lead can emerge and then suddenly vanish.

But despite that, I went on to tell my father, five areas of experimentation felt like a brief look into the near future. Neuroscientists were leaving no stone unturned. Granddad's suffering would not be in vain.

14

Regeneration

My dreams were all my own; I accounted for them to nobody; they were my refuge when annoyed – my dearest pleasure when free.

Mary Shelley, *Frankenstein*

THE YOUNG MAN peered down the microscope. The cells snapped into focus and he zoomed in. He'd spent the last ten years trying to get this experiment to work; he was getting impatient. What's more, his funding was running out and his reputation hung perilously in the balance. Maybe his colleagues were right: maybe this was a fantasy. He was, after all, hoping to rewrite the laws of nature. He steeled himself for the moment of dejection.

But it didn't come. Still he didn't know what he was looking at – but something was different. He walked away with one, all-consuming thought: *could this be it?*

Shinya Yamanaka is a smartly dressed man of mild demeanour, keen intuition and playful humour. The son of a factory owner, he grew up in Osaka, Japan, in the 1960s, and spent his childhood playing with machines before deciding to study medicine. After suffering many broken bones from rugby and judo he became interested in sports injuries and qualified as an orthopaedic surgeon. For two years he worked as a resident at Osaka National Hospital – replacing bones, resurfacing joints, repairing torn ligaments. But he soon realised his real passion lay somewhere else entirely.

In the mid-1980s biologists had started inserting genes into mouse embryos to create 'transgenic' mice. This allowed them to explore how single genes influence development and, since our genome is 99 per cent identical to that of a mouse, to explore how single genes influence human development. Yamanaka was captivated. As a surgeon the sheer number of untreatable conditions frustrated him. In this new world of molecular genetics, he realised, he could eradicate diseases by learning their underlying mechanisms. He looked for a doctoral programme that would teach him the basics of designing and executing experiments, and found one in pharmacology at Osaka City University.

After a further three years' training in America, Yamanaka returned to Japan and started generating his own mouse colony. Within six months he had 200 mice – after a year, nearly 1,000. He had to feed and clean every one himself, leaving him scant time for experiments. 'I started to think, am I really a scientist, or just a mouse keeper?'[1]

His goal was to study genes using mouse embryonic stem (ES) cells. There were two advantages to using ES cells over embryos: first, they grew and proliferated rapidly, providing a limitless supply of samples to test; second, they were pluripotent – that is, they had the potential to become any cell type in the body. By manipulating their genes Yamanaka could deduce which ones were necessary for them to become particular cell types.

But the scientists working in his department didn't see the point. 'I was often told by my colleagues, "Shinya, working on those strange mouse cells may be interesting to *you*, but perhaps you should do something more related to *medicine*."' Depressed and exhausted, Yamanaka considered quitting science altogether. But then a major event rescued him.

In 1998 a developmental biologist at the University of Wisconsin, Madison, named James Thomson, isolated the first human embryonic stem cells – the primordial material that creates an entire human being.[2] With that, a new branch of medicine, regenerative medicine, was born. Suddenly, the treatment for virtually every human disease that involved cellular and tissue deterioration was reimagined. Researchers around the world became gripped by the idea of growing made-to-order cells in a petri dish for human transplants: cardiac myocytes for heart failure, motor neurons for spinal cord injury, islet cells for diabetes, photoreceptors for blindness, and cortical neurons for Alzheimer's. And to achieve this, knowledge of how stem cells chose their cellular fate was paramount, making Yamanaka's work indispensable. He made it his mission to keep going, and was given his very own lab the following year.

As an associate professor at the Nara Institute of Science and Technology, Ikoma, Yamanaka could now begin to forge a career in science. The problem with ES cells, he soon realised, was that the patient's immune system would recognise them as foreign and mount a deadly biological defence to remove them from the body. In addition, ES cells were rapidly provoking fierce controversy due to the moral dilemma of destroying human embryos to harvest them. But the more tangible problem for Yamanaka was that he desperately needed other scientists to help kick-start his lab.

Every April, 100 students at the Nara had to select one of its twenty research labs to work for – which often left some labs with none. Students were drawn to the old, established professors, who published career-defining papers in prestigious journals like *Nature* and *Science*. At thirty-six years old, with no such papers, how, Yamanaka wondered, could he attract them? The answer came to him in a moment of breathtaking innovation.

Yamanaka wanted to test if it was possible to turn adult human cells back into stem cells – to take skin, for instance, from an individual's arm, and reprogramme it into an embryonic-like state. From this, an unlimited source of cloned human tissue could then be established. Better yet, obtained from the very person whom it was intended to help. These cells wouldn't just evade the barrier of immune rejection, they would carry the person's unique genetic signature, making them powerful tools for seeing how a patient's particular form of disease manifests. And they would be derived from adults, thereby bypassing the ethical impasse of harvesting cells from the embryo.

Not surprisingly, most scientists thought Yamanaka was dreaming. Yamanaka himself was daunted by the challenge. 'I knew how difficult it would be. It would take twenty years, thirty years, or more. But I didn't tell the students that. I just told them how wonderful it would be!' His inspired idea persuaded three students to join the lab.

They set to work. Research had already shown that stem cells required twenty-four genes to remain in a stem-like state. By artificially inserting these twenty-four genes into adult cells, Yamanaka reasoned, they might reprogramme the cells into stem cells. But using all twenty-four genes didn't work. So he tried using fewer. Again, no luck. He spent years testing various combinations of genes to see which ones were essential. 'It was like swinging a bat in pitch darkness,' he recalled. Only one student, Kazutoshi Takahashi, continued to work in the lab upon graduating. To keep Takahashi motivated, Yamanaka promised him a job for as long as he lived – so long as he kept trying to 'swing the bat'.

It worked. Just four genes, it turned out, were enough. In 2006 they demonstrated that adult cells could be reprogrammed in mice,[3] and by 2007 showed it was possible in humans as well.[4] Yamanaka called the cells 'induced pluripotent stem (iPS) cells'. He received a Nobel Prize in 2012.

In recent years, a series of landmark publications have shown that iPS cells can be turned into a host of human tissue – including liver and gut, heart, pancreas, eye and brain – paving the way for humankind to grow its own biological spare parts, and helping scientists simulate complex human diseases in a petri dish. Henceforth, the technique was aptly nicknamed 'disease-in-a-dish'.

Alzheimer's researchers had good reason to be excited about iPS cells. It represented the first step towards a wholly new kind of cure for dementia. Few organs are as inaccessible as the brain but now, for the first time, personalised neuronal cell lines from Alzheimer's patients could be developed and scrutinised. On the table were gene-editing techniques to study the effects of inserting or removing single genes; fluorescent probes to track the early signs of plaques and tangles; and even, perhaps, a cellular road map to boost cognition beyond what is natural.

As for therapeutics, their greatest strength is undoubtedly their human origin. Besides the shortcomings of mice to mirror dementia, studies also found that screening drugs in mice was far from ideal. In 2010 it was estimated that 90 per cent of drugs based on mouse models fail in clinical trials.[5] The reason: unlike mice found in the wild, lab mice are inbred, and therefore don't capture the huge genetic variation seen in people. And although their genome is very similar to ours, the way they use it – how they switch genes on and off – is very different. As the Harvard physician H. Shaw Warren put it, if one 'tried to understand a station wagon by studying a motorcycle, one would learn something about wheels and spark plugs but have no idea about steering wheels, airbags, and sunroofs, and the larger picture would be substantially missed'.[6] Indeed, one study found that only 12 per cent of the genetic changes seen in mouse models of inflammatory disorders mimicked those seen in humans[7] – providing 'a sobering reminder', wrote an editor for *Nature Methods*, 'of what most thoughtful biologists already know: your biological conclusions are really only as good as the methods that get you there'.[8]

But iPS cell modelling, too, had some troubling caveats. The reprogramming process often gave the cells strange and unpredictable characteristics. Some retained a 'memory' of their adult origins (in the form of chemical marks on their DNA) and wouldn't conform to a single population of clones. Scientists were also wary about trusting data from stem-cell-derived neurons considering neurons in Alzheimer's patients are so much older. For transplantation the concerns were more pressing: the cells might multiply uncontrollably and spawn tumours. They were also therapeutically impractical because it took roughly five months to generate them, creating the additional drawback of being extremely costly. And because the number of neurons that die in Alzheimer's is so large, scientists questioned how much iPS cell transplants could actually do; what good were they if they couldn't replace enough neurons in the time it took to harvest them? Was it even possible to grow enough? It was one thing to promise breakthroughs in the lab and quite another to translate those breakthroughs to the real world. Thankfully, many scientists believed there was little point dwelling on the obstacles, and a surge of research groups started asking patients to donate their skin.

'Yeah! Bring it on! Reimplant me!' Victoria Huntley exclaimed with a howling laugh that could probably fill a small concert hall. A professional caregiver and mother of two, she was thirty-five when she first learned of the early-onset Alzheimer's in her family. A year later, she decided to have the test. It was positive.

Victoria was one of four children born into a low-income family in Walthamstow, east London, in 1968. Growing up, she knew something wasn't right with her mother, Susan, who'd become confused, forgetful and incapable of doing simple things at home, like making a cup of tea. Before long, Susan stopped work as a hairdresser. She just couldn't do it any more: she made too many mistakes, such as giving her customers the wrong hair colour. But Susan was still in her thirties. Susan's father had died of something brain-related – he'd spent the better part of his adult life in an asylum, and Susan seemed to be heading for a similar fate. Not wanting to upset her children, she tried to hide her symptoms and carry on as normal. 'I can understand why she did that,' Victoria conceded, 'because we really were too young.'

Susan died in April 2006, when she was just fifty-six years old. In the years preceding her death, Susan's doctor's found that Susan had a rare genetic mutation in a gene named Presenilin 1 (PSEN1). Discovered in a French-Canadian family by scientists at the University of Toronto, Canada, in 1995 – four years after the APP mutation was detected – PSEN1 carriers can develop Alzheimer's as early as thirty years of age. Exactly how the gene causes such an early form of Alzheimer's remains unclear, but good evidence suggests it does so by indirectly creating plaques. That's because unlike APP (the gene for amyloid itself), PSEN1 codes for an enzyme that normally chops amyloid up into small pieces. A mutated PSEN1 therefore makes abnormally large pieces of beta-amyloid, which then clump together in the brain as plaques. And if John Hardy's amyloid cascade hypothesis is correct, that's all it takes.

In 2005, however, those kinds of particulars were the last thing on Victoria's mind. She just wanted to know if she had the PSEN1 mutation. 'Why did I want to find out?' she repeated when I put the question to her. 'Because I thought about it and thought about it, and to keep on thinking about it,' she declared, squinting her eyes in fervent concentration, 'drove me mad.' Now, although mildly symptomatic, Victoria is still able to recount how the result made her feel. 'It was the best thing I've ever done,' she told me, releasing another burst of effervescent laughter. We were chatting in her living room on a wintry November evening in 2015, her husband Martin sitting nearby, helping her remember events from the past. On Victoria's right shoulder is a tattoo of Scrabble pieces that reads: AL[. . .]HEIMER'S CAN KISS MY ARSE, the Z deliberately left blank, emphasising that something is 'missing'.

'I used to be quite a shy, sensitive person,' she continued, 'but once I found out part of me thought, *You know what, fuck it now!*' Elaborating, Martin described some of the couple's devil-may-care responses to the news since Victoria discovered what little time her mind had left. They travelled extensively – to America, Africa and the Mediterranean. They hosted big, blowout birthday parties – each year now utterly sacrosanct. And they got married; there was no point waiting any more.

When I asked what year their wedding was, Victoria couldn't remember and turned to Martin for help. He stared at the ceiling in silence for a moment too long. 'Now now!' Victoria reprimanded. 'Come on, son! Don't you slack now!'

'It was 2007,' he finally said.

'Yeah! Well done!' Victoria said. 'Well done.'

Despite their new-found insouciance, it wasn't long before the couple did start thinking about the future. After all, Victoria had two young children to consider, both with a 50 per cent chance of a strikingly abbreviated life. So when neurologists at the London Institute of Neurology asked her if she'd like to donate skin for stem cell research, she said yes without a moment's hesitation.

The Institute of Neurology occupies a twelve-storey, nondescript building not far from the British Library and the crowded underground labyrinth of King's Cross Tube station. Over 500 people work there – including Selina Wray. Growing up in the coal-mining town of Barnsley, South Yorkshire, Wray became the first in her family to go to university, and her interest in Alzheimer's stems from the inspirational mentors she had there. After her bachelor's degree in biochemistry she studied for a doctorate in the biology of Alzheimer's, and in March 2009 began work at the institute, where she now makes iPS cells from Alzheimer's patients. On 11 November 2015 I found Wray in her lab, a small windowless room containing glass beakers and pipettes, white shelves filled with chemicals and reagents, and a tall grey incubator silently inhaling carbon dioxide. A sponsorship sticker on the door reads: THIS LAB IS DEFEATING DEMENTIA.

The entire procedure is a prolonged and complicated process, involving a series of unstable, transient culture steps: an initial culture of human skin cells known as fibroblasts, made by dicing a small chunk of skin no bigger than a pea and leaving it in nutrient broth (a liquid containing essential nutrients and amino acids) for around six weeks; another fibroblast culture in which the four reprogramming genes, called Oct4, Sox2, c-Myc and Klf4 – collectively known as Yamanaka factors – are subsequently added; a three-month-long pluripotent stem cell culture, where individual fibroblasts begin to form colonies of stem cells; a neuronal precursor cell culture, composed of infant neurons which develop once the stem cells have been submerged in a special, neuron-promoting nutrient broth; and a 100-day-long period of neuronal maturation known as corticogenesis, where the neurons make synapses, fire electrical impulses, and release neurotransmitter – in this case glutamate – to finally assume a culture of adult, human, cortical glutamatergic neurons. If you're persistent enough to perform all that on a regular basis, knowing that many of your attempts will likely fail, you have a vocation for biomedical research.

A member of her team showed me some reprogrammed cells under the microscope. They looked like neurons. They behaved like neurons. They even formed synaptic contacts with each other – like neurons. It was surreal. Here, before my eyes, was a hand-made piece of someone's brain – the innermost recesses of a person's thoughts and feelings transposed onto a dish. Even after making them for seven years, Wray herself feels the same. 'When Yamanaka's discovery was out I remember thinking that it sounded a bit crazy,' she admitted. 'This idea that you could have a patient in clinic and then do all this amazing stuff just by taking a bit of their skin. I still sometimes look at them and think, wow, how is this possible?'

Each morning, Wray washes and feeds vast stockpiles of patient stem cells. If she's lucky, most will transform into neurons. But they're extremely sensitive. Indeed, every detail in the lab is designed to give them sanctuary: the incubator is set to body temperature; the fridge stocks gallons of nutrient broth; the surfaces are soaked with sterilising ethanol. On the floor sits a large yellow bin marked 'Biohazard', a final resting place for skin that didn't make the transformation.

Wray doesn't know which of her iPS cells are Victoria's; each line is strictly anonymised. She only knows some must be hers because Victoria stood up and announced her donation – with characteristic zeal – during a patient support meeting some years earlier.

Researchers are still debating how to use these neurons, but Wray's using them as a model to better understand the disease. Being this close and personal allows her to use a toolbox of molecular 'scalpels' to unveil their routine, everyday functions. By picking away at the cells' inner workings, she's able to learn how they become derailed and ultimately fatal. According to Wray, the flaws of other experimental models also define the power of iPS cells. 'The biggest disadvantage of animal models,' she explained, 'is that they don't have Alzheimer's. A mouse does *not* have Alzheimer's disease. Its brain just isn't similar enough to ours to call it that. But with iPS cells we've got the correct species, which is human, the correct cell type, which is neurons, and the correct levels of the genes we know are involved in the disease. We're mimicking the disease in real time.' But Wray has competition.

In August 2014 Doo Yeon Kim, a leading Alzheimer's researcher at Harvard University, made an embryonic stem cell culture that replicates the disease so well his model became known as Alzheimer's-in-a-dish.[9] By growing cells in a gel Kim was able to create a three-dimensional culture that looked like 'mini-spherical brains', according to one of his colleagues. Although not patient cells, these cultured neurons produced full-blown plaques and tangles in the dish, something iPS cells have yet to achieve. In fact, it was something *all* other culture models had yet to realise – beta-amyloid would just disperse in the dish, like dust, and tau never quite formed tangles. It was like trying to reproduce a Mexican gunfight without any weapons. It was described as the Achilles heel of the field. But with Kim's model, scientists could finally begin to determine what actually linked plaques to tangles on a molecular level. Moreover it offered a platform to screen hundreds of thousands of drugs in a matter of months.

But Wray isn't fazed. 'I think both models actually complement each other,' she said. 'It's just about choosing the model most appropriate to the scientific question you're asking.'

So what was Victoria's PSEN1 mutation telling scientists like Wray? 'Everything we're seeing makes a strong case to support the amyloid cascade hypothesis,' she said. 'But I think we have to target both amyloid and tau, because once the disease starts I think tau takes over. And why not do both: block disease initiation but still assume some tangles have already formed?'

And what about transplantation? Did she think it would eventually be possible to make new neurons in the dish and then reinsert those into a dementing brain? 'I think never say never, because even the development of this technology took everyone by surprise. But I'm inclined to think that that's not where their strength lies. When you look at an Alzheimer's brain post-mortem the loss of cells is so vast and widespread. So to take these cells and put them back and then expect them to integrate into the kind of brain circuitry that was there before . . . it's too big an ask, I think. At the moment anyway.'

That 'ask' pivots on finding a solution to two problems. The first is a structural problem. Born from the outer skin of the embryo, the brain undergoes a series of complex steps to reach maturity, unfolding in an exquisitely delicate process of timing and precision. Because Alzheimer's undoes this so ruthlessly, iPS cell technology may have to reach a stage where scientists can grow whole sections of brain – replete with blood vessels, myelin and cerebrospinal fluid – to achieve meaningful results upon transplantation. (It's why Kim's mini-spherical brains are so encouraging.) The second problem is one of integration. The brain takes a long time to grow. Many of the genes responsible for setting it up are only activated during key windows of development in the first few years of life; conversely, certain genes lie dormant until adulthood. So unless scientists can engineer iPS cells to better reflect such molecular fine-tuning, transplanting them could be, as a professor once put it, like asking an amateur pianist to play Chopin's last ballade.

Nevertheless, there are hints that transplantation might work. In 2014 Penelope Hallett of Harvard University did a post-mortem on patients who, fourteen years earlier, had received stem cell grafts for Parkinson's disease (another affliction involving catastrophic neuronal loss). Amazingly, Hallett found that not only did the grafts remain healthy and intact, they matured and integrated in the host brain as well.[10] A year later, she went further, exploring how implantation might actually work in practice. The procedure is known as autogenic stem cell transplantation (auto-SCT): a technique where an injection of iPS cells physically engrafts the cells into the required bodily location. And the reality isn't far off. Using primate models of Parkinson's, Hallett's team has shown that auto-SCT of iPS cells taken from the skin can partially rebuild the substantia nigra, the brain region destroyed by Parkinson's disease. This improved the animals' movement symptoms for up to two years.

Other data suggests that stem cells needn't engraft at all. Rather, their mere presence may help by providing restorative, 'neurotrophic' support to diseased brain regions. That was illustrated in 2009 at the University of California, Irvine, when Frank LaFerla injected stem cells into the brain of Alzheimer's transgenic mice.[11] Within a month the animals' memory improved. And yet, the stem cells didn't turn into neurons. Or have any impact on plaques and tangles. Instead, they were quietly churning out the protein BDNF (brain-derived neurotrophic factor), which alone was enough to boost synapse density in the hippocampus by 67 per cent.

Still, Wray's concerns are echoed by many in the field. On 6 November 2014 stem cell biologists from all over the world amassed in Durham, North Carolina, for a conference titled, 'Accelerating the cure for Alzheimer's disease through regenerative medicine'. The topic under discussion was whether stem cells – both iPS and embryonic – are ready to enter clinical trials as transplants. The audience included delegates from biotech and Big Pharma, as well as senior academics. And feelings were mixed. Some said the technology was still a long way from being safe, let alone effective. Only two months had passed since Masayo Takahashi, an ophthalmologist in Kobe, Japan, had to abandon her efforts to implant iPS-derived retinal cells into the right eye of a woman with macular degeneration, when Yamanaka spotted two potentially carcinogenic mutations in her batch; giving this woman cancer in an attempt to correct her sight would have been disastrous. There were more fundamental uncertainties regarding Alzheimer's. It still wasn't known where to deliver the cells, for instance, or how many were needed, and how often. And would they have any impact on plaques and tangles? No one knew.

But others stressed that clinical trials inform research just as much as research informs clinical trials; indeed, scientists could spend years mulling over uncertainties and still have the same basic concerns. And so phase one clinical trials are now being discussed, marking the first, tentative steps in a new era of brain regeneration.

This is all too late for Victoria, of course. But she's accepted that with remarkable resilience and unwavering altruism. 'I know what's going to happen . . . but there's nothing I can . . . do . . . about it . . .' Eight months had passed since my first visit and she was unmistakably worse: less animated, more introverted, she strained to vocalise her thoughts. 'So I just hope . . . they find something . . . for somebody else.' Her memory had taken a nose-dive, said Martin. She now forgot what she was doing from one moment to the next. Times, dates and day-to-day norms like shopping or going for walks were fast becoming incomprehensible. One day, Martin found that she'd unwittingly put cutlery in the bin; on another, he observed her hysterically searching for her phone while holding it in her hand all along. Martin, now a bulwark of patience and fortitude, has adapted; he's 'just been getting on with it', he said.

Given Victoria's condition, I was amazed to hear that she'd recently resumed her old job. Every few weeks she's taken to see an old friend, called Iris, who suffers from Alzheimer's herself. Victoria met Iris more than a decade ago, when she worked as a carer. She'd nursed Iris's daughter, who had Down's syndrome, and was now doing what little she could to see Iris, a ninety-one-year-old, through the final stages of a fate she knows awaits her too. She told me that she was bored at home; that she wanted to keep her mind active. 'I've always been in the caring game,' she said proudly, 'but . . . of course . . . I'm know I can't make . . . any mistakes . . . and I . . .' She trailed off and Martin filled in the blanks. For him, the undertaking was not so much to keep Victoria occupied as it was to give her some company while he's at work. His intuition is well founded: studies show that staying socially active can relieve anxiety and depression in dementia.

Wanting to offer something, anything, I relayed some of the

dazzling work being done using her cells in the lab – impossible were it not for Victoria's contribution. I still found it hard to digest the knowledge that while Victoria's mind slowly deconstructs, it was quietly being reconstructed under the nose of Wray and other scientists, creating a portal to somewhere no brain scan can go. It's hard to say when expectation will meet reality for iPS cells. There is a huge element of luck in biological research. Take Louis Pasteur, the French pioneer of vaccination. His discovery of the chicken cholera vaccine only occurred when he abandoned the experiment out of frustration and took a vacation, returning to discover that leaving the broth was precisely what was necessary to 'attenuate', or weaken, the bacteria enough for it to become a vaccine. This kind of thing happens all the time in modern laboratories. It comes from the sheer lawlessness of biology, the 'most lawless of the three basic sciences', wrote cancer biologist Siddhartha Mukherjee. 'There are few rules to begin with, and even fewer rules that are universal.'[12]

Nowhere else is this truer than in cell biology. We can imagine cells as microcosms of modern megacities – dynamic, ever-changing entities, constantly generating new and innovative trends in behaviour. With iPS cells, it's like finding a city on another planet. And so for the time being, the nitty-gritty of how they actually work is a total enigma. Scientists are basically making it up as they go along.

Nevertheless, some exciting practical developments are emerging. In the decade since Yamanaka unveiled them, iPS cells have been made from hair follicles and even urine. Researchers have envisioned iPS cell 'banks', stockpiling varieties that would be compatible for the wider population. This has piqued the interest of the US Department of Defense, which is now funding research to create self-renewing banks of red blood cells for injured soldiers in combat; according to one estimate, only forty donors of varying blood types would be needed to supply the general population indefinitely.[13] Outbreaks of tropical infections such as Zika are also reaping the benefits. Researchers at Johns Hopkins University in Baltimore, Maryland, recently used iPS cells to determine how the Zika infection in pregnant women may cause microcephaly, a birth defect in which a baby's head is smaller than usual.[14] In the future we can imagine even more far-reaching applications. As one expert told *Nature*'s Megan Scudellari in June 2016: 'The world is watching . . .'[15]

For evidence that even more incredible feats of regeneration are being pursued, one need look no further than the morbid and fascinating events that unfolded in California in the spring of 2012.

15

Young Blood

And so we remained till the red of the dawn began to fall through the snow gloom. I was desolate and afraid, and full of woe and terror. But when that beautiful sun began to climb the horizon life was to me again.

Bram Stoker, *Dracula*

IN 1956, HALF a century before Yamanaka's work galvanised the concept of regenerative medicine, a gerontologist at Cornell University called Clive McCay performed a ghoulish experiment. Using small scissors and surgical sutures, he stitched together pairs of rats – one young and one old – making their circulatory systems unite.[1] It was called parabiosis (from the Greek *para*, meaning 'alongside', and *bios*, for 'life'), and was done to investigate 'the possibility,' he wrote, 'of reversing the pathological changes in an old animal by bathing its tissue in the blood of a young one'.

McCay's work extended that of the German alchemist Andreas Libavius, who in 1615 proposed joining the arteries of an old man to those of a young one. While it was never determined if Libavius actually carried out the experiment, he evidently had strong convictions about its efficacy, concluding that 'the hot and spirituous blood of the young man will pour into the old one as if it were from a fountain of youth, and all of his weakness will be dispelled'.[2]

French zoologist Paul Bert was inspired by Libavius, and in 1864, using rats, he published a radical study – 'Expériences et considérations sur la greffe animale' – that became the earliest recorded parabiosis experiment.[3] It won him an award from the French Academy of Sciences. Bert's aim, though, was principally to demonstrate the method's feasibility; he showed that veins formed between the two rats, and that fluid injected into one animal passed into the vein of the other.

But McCay had the same inclinations as Libavius, and was obsessed with unlocking the biological mechanisms of ageing and longevity. Since antiquity, ageing had been attributed to the decline of a mysterious factor the Greeks called 'innate heat', which, when extinguished, left the body cold and dry. And for millennia there have been tales of a fabled 'Fountain of Youth', which gives everlasting youth to those who drink from its waters. Throughout history, there have also been rumours that the mysterious elixir of youth resides in young blood. The Roman emperor Constantine was reputedly advised by pagan priests to bathe in the blood of children to cure his leprosy. When children went missing in Paris in the 1700s, it was thought that King Louis XV was bathing in their blood. It was even rumoured that the late North Korean dictator Kim Jong-Il tried to slow down his own ageing by injecting himself with the blood of healthy young virgins.

These gruesome, extraordinary tales just might have a rational basis despite the horrifying crimes some of them suggest. In his experiments, McCay found that the constant exchange of blood between old and young rats made the bones of the older animals similar in strength to those of their young partners. Something in the blood was rejuvenating them, but what was it? And what else might it revive? For reasons that aren't entirely clear, though perhaps due to its dark implications, the work was scarcely followed up. It wasn't until recently that two US universities started to provide answers.

The first was a Harvard University group led by Amy Wagers, an ambitious stem cell biologist with dusty blonde hair and grey-blue eyes. Wagers resurrected parabiosis while training under Irving Weissman at Stanford University in the early 2000s. Weissman had spent decades studying examples of parabiosis in nature and was fascinated by a sea-dwelling creature called the Star Ascidian (which reproduces as a bud, grows off its parent, and remains joined to it until the parent eventually dies and is reabsorbed by the offspring). When Wagers expressed an interest in exploring the movement of circulating blood stem cells, Weissman advised her to use parabiotic mice. She pursued the work at Harvard, where she established her own laboratory in May 2004.

Back at Stanford, word spread of the spooky method Wagers was employing for her experiments, and it wasn't long before researchers interested in the biology of ageing, led by a neurologist called Thomas Rando, asked her to work alongside them. Wagers agreed, flew back to Stanford, and in 2005 the team discovered that joining young and old mice rejuvenates muscle and liver tissue in older animals.[4]

At Harvard, Wagers then went on to show that young blood could even rejuvenate the heart and spinal cord. It was flabbergasting; all the ancient folklore about the merits of young blood suddenly had scientific endorsement. It sparked a media sensation. One headline read: VAMPIRE THERAPY: YOUNG BLOOD MAY REVERSE AGEING.[5]

Inspired by Wagers's findings, another Stanford neurologist named Tony Wyss-Coray decided to take things further, and investigate if young blood had any bearing on people with Alzheimer's.

In a single day, human blood travels through 96,000 kilometres of capillaries, veins and arteries – enough to encircle the globe four times. It passes through every organ in the body, but a hefty 25 per cent of its volume flows solely through the brain. Why? Because it's doing a lot more than ferrying oxygen. Besides red and white blood cells, blood carries more than 700 proteins in its plasma, the fluid portion of blood. What many of them do is completely unknown. But like everything else, they change as we age: some fade away while others appear more. What, then, asked Wyss-Coray, might those changes mean for the brain, and could they affect memory?

To find answers, Wyss-Coray began by using blood plasma from young mice. First, he set up a unique type of water maze that tests spatial memory. Known as the Morris water maze, the animal is placed in a pool of water and can only escape by swimming around until it remembers the location of a small hidden platform. A young mouse will usually find the platform quickly, whereas older animals struggle to remember its whereabouts and thus take longer (it's a bit like trying to find your car in a busy car park after a long day of shopping). Remarkably, when Wyss-Coray injected young plasma into old mice they fared just as well in the maze as their younger counterparts.[6]

Emboldened, Wyss-Coray moved on to investigate what was occurring at the cellular level. In mammals, especially humans, learning and memory are linked to brain circuits found in the cerebral cortex and hippocampus. The number and strength of cells in these regions – strength here being LTP, the neural analogue of memory I discussed in chapter three – essentially determines how good these higher cognitive faculties are. And so, after performing parabiosis on pairs of old–young mice, Wyss-Coray got his team to stain thin slices of their brain tissue with a dye that binds new-born neurons. Amazingly, the older mice had three to four times as many new neurons in their hippocampus as their younger counterparts. What's more, the young mice showed the opposite effect, displaying a stunted birth of neurons instead. Wyss-Coray then decided to focus on the dentate gyrus, an area of the hippocampus that regulates the formation of new memories. What he found stunned him. The neurons in the older animals were generating more synapses and demonstrating enhanced LTP. Their memories were improving. And the younger animals, again, showed the exact opposite.

Why was this happening? He suspected it had something to do with how neurons are born in the adult brain. In the developing brain, the birth of new neurons – dubbed neurogenesis – is highly active. It was once thought neurogenesis is restricted to the embryo, until research in the 1980s showed it also occurs in adults via a population of adult stem cells known as neural stem cells (NSCs).

The hippocampus is one of the few brain regions where nurseries of NSCs reside. These nurseries, it turns out, also happen to live right next to blood vessels. And that got Wyss-Coray thinking.

In an earlier paper he had noted that 'diminished neurogenesis during ageing may be modulated by the balance of two independent forces: intrinsic [brain]–derived cues, and cues extrinsic to the [brain] delivered by blood'.[7] So what was it about old blood that had such profound *anti*-neurogenesis effects? To find out, he compared over sixty different blood proteins between old and young mice, and one protein stood out. It was called eotaxin, and it was far more abundant in older animals. It belonged to a family of molecules known to have roles in brain development and, strangely, asthma. Beyond that, not much was known about it. To rule out the chance that increased eotaxin was harmless, Wyss-Coray injected the protein into young mice, only to get the same results: decreased neurogenesis, decreased LTP, impaired learning and memory in the water maze.

That was in 2011, and the results seemed too good to be true. Indeed, when the group first submitted the work for publication the reviewers rejected it on that very basis. So the scientists spent a year repeating the experiments at a different facility. Again, the data checked out. And so, by 2012, Wyss-Coray started investigating what was happening at the genetic level.

In the aged animals, young blood was activating a master gene called CREB. Since the early 1990s, CREB had been well known for its clear role in stabilising long-term memories. Exactly how it does that isn't clear, but good evidence suggests it does so by controlling how other genes are activated. But whatever the mechanism, the discovery plainly showed that young blood has a deep and powerful effect on memory. Wyss-Coray published those findings in June 2014, and they immediately hit the press. The authors suddenly found themselves having to turn down lucrative requests from old-aged billionaires, exclusive invitations to celebrity dinner parties, and, of course, a deluge of emails from patient relatives, imploring them to test it on their loved ones.

It could have ended there – with Wyss-Coray's team mining

blood, imaging hippocampi and timing mice in the water maze. After all, they still had a kaleidoscopic range of blood proteins to investigate. But a chance encounter with the grandson of a Chinese businessman made them drastically reconsider their next step.

Mr Li Wei was ten years old when he left school to work for a silk merchant. The eldest son of a destitute family in the Zhejiang province of mainland China, his starving siblings gave him little choice. In his early teens he moved to Shanghai and worked his way into a position where he became the protégé of wealthy investors and business tycoons, learning everything he could so that he might one day return home to save his family. By the age of twenty, he had helped get his father's dying textile business back on its feet, and by twenty-six had moved to Hong Kong to start his very own cotton-spinning factory. That was in 1949. Today, his company is worth just shy of $5 billion.

During his life, Li expanded his business into real estate, shipping and finance, gave generously to Buddhist charities and philanthropic organisations, got married, and raised two daughters. According to his grandson, Alex, now in his early thirties, he was an intense, energetic man who slept only four hours a night, shunned holidays and hobbies, and saw making money more like a game than making a living. 'Working was his life,' said Alex, sitting opposite me in a conference room on the top floor of the company's Hong Kong skyscraper. Below and across the street lay Victoria Harbour, with the frenetic mix of tower blocks, designer brands, teahouses and temples of Kowloon beyond. 'He was our role model, the foundation of all we have. So seeing his decline was painful.'

The family first suspected something wasn't right when Li started becoming unusually aggressive during family dinners. Looking back, they think that was some time in the late 1990s; it's hard to give an exact date, because Li was so passionate about work that for a while the family thought he was simply having bad days at the office. But by the mid-2000s it was obvious. Gaping holes in Li's short- and long-term memory emerged; suddenly, he couldn't remember where he had been the previous night, or the names of fellow business associates he'd worked with for years. His one and only pastime of Xiangqi (Chinese chess) was becoming a total enigma; unwittingly, he started making up his own rules to compensate. Terrified at the prospect of losing the man Alex described as their 'Superman', the family employed a group of private nurses and looked into every available treatment.

This was done quietly. In China, and many other Far Eastern Asian nations, Alzheimer's is still deeply stigmatised. 'The Chinese translation for Alzheimer's is something along the lines of "elderly retardation disease",' Alex confessed, while his assistant poured us a glass of warm water (a Chinese tradition). 'Recently it's been renamed "regression of the brain" disease, but it's always been a taboo. And nursing homes are not very popular here, because to the Chinese you really are supposed to take care of your parents until they pass. Putting them in a nursing home is almost viewed as an irresponsible act.'

For years the family struggled to hide Li's condition from outsiders, afraid of what people – especially his business partners – would think. But in 2009 something extraordinary forced them to speak out. Li, then aged eighty-six, was coming to the final stages of Alzheimer's. He slept most of the day, was spoon-fed, scarcely recognised his family, and was in and out of hospital for other medical conditions. During one such hospital visit, he received a blood plasma transfusion as part of a routine procedure. The result was miraculous.

'Before the transfusion he didn't say anything; he was like a child of one or two years old,' Alex explained. 'After, however, he looked at my mom and said, "I want to go home."'

'She said, "Okay, let me call the chauffeur."'

'Then he said, "Okay fine, let's go downstairs and wait for him."'

'To which my mom said, "Why don't you just wait here, because the nurses might be coming."'

'And he replied, "Okay, why don't we do this: *you* wait here, and I will wait downstairs for the car."'

'They were having a dialogue!' Alex exclaimed in disbelief. 'He was *negotiating*. To us, that was a huge jump.'

It didn't end there. Li remembered old faces and old staff members. He even spoke to them about business and current affairs. He experienced moments of 'pure lucidity', said Alex, which lasted as long as four days. It wasn't much, but for the family, that felt like an eternity.

It was no fluke, either. Li had the procedure a further three times and each time yielded a similar result. The hospital doctors were baffled. They didn't want to explicitly say that Li's improvements were caused by the young plasma, lest they give a potentially false sense of hope. So Li's family gratefully accepted what they'd been given, and surreptitiously documented the events should a time come when it might prove useful. They knew nothing of the experiments going on in America – until, one day in spring 2013, Alex decided to share the story with a family friend and scientist named Karoly Nikolich.

'I immediately told him about Tony Wyss-Coray's work,' Nikolich said, sitting in his home office in Palo Alto, California. I'd just asked him to recount the inception of this radical new therapy, and he was beaming. It was 5 a.m. for him – the time he usually starts his day – and we were talking over Skype. He was easy-going and casually dressed, and yet had the face of a stern industrialist. 'Afterwards I rang Tony and said, "Can you believe this!?" He said it was the first time he'd ever heard of a human situation where this may actually be helpful. We were fascinated.'

Alex had told the Hungarian professor about his grandfather over lunch in Hong Kong. Though Nikolich worked primarily at Stanford, he also acted as a scientific adviser for the family's occasional investment forays in biotechnology. Soon after their conversation, the pair started brainstorming over how best to move forward. A government-funded trial was out of the question: funding was hard enough to come by as it was, let alone funding for something based on the anecdotal observations of a single patient. So

Alex agreed to fund it himself, providing $3 million for Nikolich and Wyss-Coray to establish their very own company. They called it Alkahest, after the mythical substance that chemists in the fifteenth century thought had the power to cure all disease.

Since January 2014, Alkahest has enrolled a small number of people with mild to moderate Alzheimer's. 'So far we've done about sixty infusions,' Nikolich revealed to me, 'and we haven't seen any adverse effects. This isn't an official report, but I think we're comfortable with the safety.' Understandably, he was reluctant to tell me whether they had actually seen any cognitive improvements. Optimism can be a dangerous thing in science. There's already a black market for body organs, and Wyss-Coray now gets emails from people offering to bleed children for his research. But the pair have a more basic concern at the moment – supply. A simple calculation shows that the entire planet's young plasma supply would only be enough for 3 per cent of the world's Alzheimer's patients.

Alkahest's ultimate goal, therefore, is a pill containing purified blood proteins. It may only take a few; Nikolich thinks three to five proteins should do the job. But before he continued, my impatience got the better of me.

'How long?' I asked.

He smiled. 'It's too early to say.'

Unsatisfied with that answer, I did more research and discovered that others have put it at fifteen to twenty years. I almost wished I hadn't looked. There's a maddening quality to being both a scientist and a patient relative. One part of you knows to leave emotion out of it; the other is furious at the sheer indifference of when nature chooses to reveal its secrets. But I found something else while digging, too. In early 2015 a Spanish chemical company called Grifols put nearly $40 million into Alkahest for a 45 per cent share in the company. Victor Grifols, the company's eponymous CEO, announced that the collaboration would finally address 'the major unmet medical need of this century'. I made a note to call the company in one year's time – and every year thereafter.

In the meantime, I was eager to hear Nikolich's thoughts on

what caused Alzheimer's. He'd taken such a left-field approach to curing the malady, I wondered if he could even class himself as a Bapist, Tauist, or E4ist.

'I'm not in any camp, actually. My gut feeling is that this probably has deeper roots.' Wanting to offer me something constructive, he leaned back in his chair and rummaged through a nearby bookshelf, pulling out books and papers by other unconventional thinkers. He told me about a group in Seattle, Washington, who are studying brain ageing in domestic dogs – the rationale being that because dogs share our living space and also succumb to dementia, they may hold a clue that mice and humans do not. He also spoke about a substance found in the soil of Easter Island by Canadian scientists in 1964, called Rapamycin, which has been shown to extend the lifespan of mice by 14 per cent.[8]

Amid all these arresting developments, though, Nikolich stressed a crucial message: the mission, he said, is extended *healthspan*, not lifespan. Because even if we all live to 150, 'nobody wants to live long as a vegetable,' he bluntly concluded.

But some believe this is a false dichotomy. Aubrey de Grey, an eccentric computer scientist and gerontologist at Cambridge University, thinks the only way to extend healthspan is by radically extending human lifespan. Repairing the molecular damage of ageing, he claims, should eventually allow us to live healthy lives well into our hundreds if not thousands. Adults could be sixty chronologically, but remain in their thirties biologically. As the technology advances the gap would then stretch out over centuries, with the knock-on effect of eradicating all age-related diseases – including Alzheimer's. In *Ending Aging: The Rejuvenation Breakthroughs That Could Reverse Human Aging in Our Lifetime*, de Grey predicts a time when

> we might take a regular sequence of anti-amyloid vaccines, not unlike the standardized series now given in regular succession over the course of our childhood; we would get a 'booster shot' of some every few years, while others would be administered only a few times in each century of a greatly expanded lifespan. Each time we

took one of these vaccines, our cells and organs would once again live and function free of a specific species of molecular bindweeds [i.e. plaques and tangles], returning them to the literally *unbound* potential of youth.[9]

Approaching seventy himself, Nikolich admitted that healthy ageing is fast becoming his obsession. But his memory is as good as ever: through the bright glow of my computer screen, he recalled the hardships of growing up in a communist satellite of the Soviet bloc, and how his parents had to scrape together makeshift chemistry sets to better educate him about science and the wider world. Now, it seemed, fate had put him, Li Wei and Wyss-Coray together to revive and realise an ancient fantasy.

On a less grandiose note, there's a plain and important lesson to be learned from the events of this chapter, aptly stated by Alex before I left him in Hong Kong. 'For us, this was really just an observation of my grandfather. If every caretaker of patients who've been through medical procedures could just document things more, that's already a significant step. And it's simple, right?'

In the rigorous, dispassionate realm of academia, anecdotal evidence is often given short shrift. It suffers mainly from having no experimental 'control' – no objective means of comparison, that is – to minimise variables and increase scientific objectivity. We depend on controls to infer whether two things are causally linked. But as Alex and Li have demonstrated, anecdotes sometimes have another power. They can lead to new hypotheses. They can take what seems absurd and use it to arouse creativity. No one would seriously consider bleeding the young to restore the old. And yet, something valuable was hiding within such an absurdity all along. It just took a perceptive relative to shake it loose.

16

Seeds of Dementia

The fox knows many things,
but the hedgehog knows one big thing.
                    Archilochus, Greek proverb

B Y THE TIME I finished my doctorate at University College
London, half the scientists in the department were entranced
by a new lead. When I first heard about it, though, I felt a
troubling coalescing of intrigue and dread. Naturally we all had
our own pet hypothesis about what caused Alzheimer's. It was not
unusual for a group of us to meet in the kitchen over tea or coffee
and quiz each other about our respective ideas; such encounters
were welcome and – for the most part – civil. But something about
this one went too far. It made us question everything we thought
we knew. Whether that was reasonable scepticism or insecure pride,
I don't know. But when I buttonholed one of its advocates boiling
the kettle one day, and forced him to explain it to me, the story
he told almost made me want to wear a hazmat suit to work.

Deep in the tropical rainforest of Papua New Guinea, in the Okapa
region along the Eastern Highlands above the Lamari River, lies a
row of small, thatched huts lashed together by bamboo stems and
grass. It's a village called Agakamatasa. Few go there. It's home to
a prehistoric tribe called the Fore: a tribe that once, according
to anthropologists, indulged in ritualistic cannibalism.

But in March 1957 an American paediatrician called Carleton

Gajdusek did go there. Gajdusek was thirty-three, a workaholic with lively blue eyes and a renowned love of conversation. (Once, when asked before a lecture if he was nervous, he replied, 'No, I am only nervous when I am not talking.') The son of a Slovakian butcher, he grew up in New York and studied at Harvard, where his charismatic energy earned him the nickname 'atom bomb'. Soon tiring of American life, Gajdusek elected to pursue infectious diseases in primitive cultures. As an army medic he travelled the globe to study rabies, plague, scurvy and haemorrhagic fevers. It wasn't long before he heard about the Fore tribe in New Guinea, who were suffering from a mysterious illness they named kuru, a word meaning 'to shake'.

Kuru wasn't pleasant. Its victims suffered wild spasms and slurred speech, followed by ominous fits of laughter, which culminated in a slow, sometimes year-long, gut-wrenching demise. The ruling Australian government called it the Laughing Death. It affected nearly 200 people a year, threatening to eradicate the roughly 35,000 Fore altogether. They believed kuru was the work of sorcerers from rival tribes; some would even hire local counter-sorcerers to fend off the illness with chants and protective herbs. Gajdusek, however, was eager to discover the real cause, and so decided to move to Agakamatasa and stay a while.

He established a makeshift laboratory in a large, circular hut, gathered as many samples as he could, and performed post-mortems. Though wary of his curious instruments and outlandish concepts, the Fore grew fond of Gajdusek. They called him 'Doctor America'.

Because kuru mainly affected movement, Gajdusek tracked its source to the brain – where, sure enough, something was terribly wrong. It was freckled with numerous sponge-like holes. Perplexed, Gajdusek shipped some samples to his colleagues. Despite being similarly mystified by its cause, they were struck by its resemblance to Creutzfeldt-Jakob disease (CJD), the human form of 'mad cow disease'. CJD is a freakish, fatal condition that usually arises spon-taneously in people's sixties. It causes a rapid loss of memory and cognition, abnormal movements and muscle stiffness, visual problems and slurred speech, and most patients lapse into a coma and die within a year. But kuru also bore an uncanny likeness to scrapie, a disease that caused sheep to shake and compulsively scrape their skin against trees or fences.

It turned out that all three afflictions were transmissible: CJD could pass from person to person during medical procedures; scrapie infected other sheep by close contact; and kuru, they realised, was spread by cannibalism. Since 1890 the Fore had staged funeral rituals where family members were cooked and eaten. Nothing was wasted – especially the brain, which they considered the seat of the soul. Eating it, they believed, gave the dead eternal life. But what was the infectious agent? A virus? A bacterium? Perhaps some kind of parasite? It had to be one, but the evidence was non-existent.

The truth, when it arrived twenty years later, was a scientific heresy that changed our view of Alzheimer's for ever.

It came from a neurologist named Stanley Prusiner. Prusiner was not a popular man: during the mid-1980s, at the defining point of his career, he was called 'impulsive', 'presumptuous', 'reckless', 'aggressive', 'manipulative' and 'egotistical'. But Prusiner uncovered something that baffled some and downright incensed others. The agent for kuru, CJD and scrapie was not a micro-organism: it was a protein, an infectious one that survived and reproduced without DNA – violating every rule in the book.

Prusiner dubbed these weird new particles 'prions', a tweaked portmanteau of *pro*tein and *in*fection (in fact prions were so weird, they later became the inspiration for Kurt Vonnegut's 'Ice-nine' – an infectious crystal that kills by hardening the body's water into ice – in his science fiction novel *Cat's Cradle*). Most disturbingly, Prusiner soon discovered that healthy brains make prions all the time. The only reason everyone didn't have kuru or CJD was because prions live a shadowy double life. In normal brain cells a prion is harmless and actually has a function: according to recent evidence, it helps insulate neurons. But every so often a neuron will accidentally manufacture a prion with a deformed three-dimensional shape. A protein with a deformed shape is as useless as a mangled house key. Usually our cells spot these biochemical mishaps and either refold the protein into its normal shape or, failing that, destroy it.

But somehow, in the brains of those with kuru, the prion's deformed rogue twin evades these fail-safe mechanisms. Worse, it then corrupts copies of normal prions until they too become deadly rogue twins. If enough normal prions are recruited this way, a chain reaction ensues, and pernicious hordes of prions rise and spread like cancer. That prions are capable of this without using DNA is baffling because every other known infectious agent needs a genome to construct fresh copies of itself.

The existence of such an insidious entity was deeply concerning. More unnerving, however, were the similarities between prion infections and Alzheimer's. In the early 1990s a German anatomist named Heiko Braak looked at thousands of patient brains and described how beta-amyloid and tau spread through the brain in a strikingly prion-like fashion.[1] Tangles start at the base of the brain, he said, then creep into the hippocampus before eventually fanning out to the rest of the cortex. Plaques do the same, only in the opposite direction. It was almost as if Alzheimer's had been seeded.

And there was more. During his training, Prusiner met a patient called George Balanchine. The founder of the New York City Ballet, Balanchine was a renowned choreographer and ballet master but began complaining of 'unsteadiness' in September 1978. Before long his balance problems worsened and he started to experience severe memory loss and confusion. By February 1983 he was unable to speak and died one month later. A post-mortem finally revealed the cause. It was CJD. But bewilderingly, Balanchine's brain was filled with dark clumps of protein, just like the plaques seen in the brains of Alzheimer's patients.

It begged a question with huge implications: is Alzheimer's a prion disease? Prusiner thought about this for a long time. He knew the possibility of Alzheimer's being something one could 'catch' was highly unlikely, because attempts to transmit it from humans to animals had proved unsuccessful.

Until 2006, that is.

Mathias Jucker told me he's wary of speaking to the public about his work. He doesn't want to cause alarm. Alzheimer's is *not* infectious, he stressed, and the best way for me to understand the prion link was to imagine dominoes. 'When the first domino falls, the others fall too. The seed is the first domino,' he asserted in his deep German accent. 'And I want to catch it before it falls.'

Jucker is handsome and athletic-looking, with short grey hair and a marvellous excess of candour. In September 2006, on the hundredth anniversary of Alzheimer's ill-famed lecture, and only a short train ride from the notorious Frankfurt asylum, Jucker reported a shocking new transmission of the substance that plagued Auguste Deter all those years ago. Taking brain tissue from deceased Alzheimer's patients, Jucker injected it into the brains of young mice and then waited to see if anything happened. Within four months, seeds of beta-amyloid had sown in the hippocampus, before spreading – like weeds – to other parts of the animals' brains.[2] They were behaving just like prions. 'We'd long anticipated that other proteins would behave like prions, so we just looked at what the prion people were doing and did the same,' Jucker explained, as if it were obvious. His desire to understand how amyloid seeds function like prions is not merely academic; it will help to design small molecules that can stop the proteins dead in their tracks. 'Mouse hosts are good because they allow us to do the experiment fast. But now everyone's trying to find out what the initial seed is in humans. And the idea of an initial seed is a beautiful thing to say to the public, because if it's true I could just develop antibodies and make sure that I get rid of this one seed. But of course, it might be that there's more than one; that many dominoes can fall at the same time.'

Jucker's primary obstacle is a pitfall all researchers must face: the divide between *in vitro* and *in vivo*, Latin for 'within the glass' and 'within the living', respectively. *In vitro* is good for scrutinising nature at the microscopic level; single molecules surrender their secrets far more readily when isolated from the body, a system so complex it often drowns out meaningful data with background noise. But there's a catch: the very act of isolating such molecules can change their behaviour. And so that *in vitro* clue – which in Jucker's case takes the form of beta-amyloid seeds extracted from post-mortem brain tissue – may in fact be a perversion of what's actually happening in the living brain. It's arguably the biggest hurdle facing drug developers. If it were easy to surmount, 'drug discovery would be as reliable as drug manufacturing,' notes Pfizer Pharmaceuticals veteran Christopher Lipinski.[3]

Since 2006 Jucker has been trying to extrapolate his findings to living humans by searching for beta-amyloid seeds in bodily fluids. His team had got proof it was a lead worth chasing when, in November 2010, they showed that injecting beta-amyloid into a mouse's belly triggered plaque formation in the brain.[4] It took five months and appeared to have created tangles to boot. How this happened, they don't know. It's possible the seeds were ferried into the brain through some undiscovered cell-to-cell transport mechanism. If proven, that will be a serious blow to stem cell research, for how can a stem cell therapy ever succeed if seeds of beta-amyloid can circle the body like vultures, waiting to inflict dementia all over again?

If Jucker does identify the first falling domino (or dominoes), as he so eloquently puts it, a Nobel Prize is on the cards. Meanwhile, a few inconvenient truths kept the question of Alzheimer's prion ancestry alive. For one thing, different strains of prions cause different prion diseases, all of which display a wide variety of symptoms; it's possible, therefore, that different 'strains' of beta-amyloid and tau account for variations in the symptoms of Alzheimer's sufferers. For another, Jucker's breakthrough coincided with a breakthrough by a group of Cambridge University researchers, who had demonstrated Alzheimer's transmission in primates – a mammal uncomfortably close to us.[5] And so, feverishly, scientists persevered at unlocking the connection. Thankfully, human-to-human transmission of Alzheimer's pathology had never been seen.

What happened next almost caused a serious public health scare. Reporting in the September 2015 issue of *Nature*, John Collinge, a world-renowned prion researcher at University College London, offered the first evidence that beta-amyloid may very well be transmitted between people.[6] His team were investigating the brains of eight people who'd died from CJD. Aged between thirty-six and fifty-four, the patients had received pituitary growth hormone thirty years earlier; it was a routine treatment for children with dwarfism or stunted growth. Until 1985 the hormone was sourced from human cadavers. An estimated 30,000 children were treated with cadaveric growth hormone and most lived – and are living – full, healthy lives at a normal height. But a small percentage of children contracted the lethal prion disease during surgery. The tragedy was especially common in France, where surgeons unwittingly used older cadavers, more likely to be reservoirs of prions because the risk of CJD increases with age. As a consequence, 125 children died – and in a Parisian courtroom in October 2010 two French doctors narrowly avoided charges of involuntary manslaughter.[7]

As if the hormone recipients' problems weren't bad enough, Collinge found that six of the eight brains under scrutiny were also teeming with beta-amyloid. How had this happened? None had any genes for early-onset Alzheimer's, nor were they old enough to have so much amyloid in their brains. The most plausible explanation, according to Collinge, is that the protein 'piggybacked' its way in on the growth hormone during their injections. Worryingly, he might be right. Beta-amyloid sticks to metal like industrial glue, and unlike bacteria or viruses, you can boil, bake, desiccate and even irradiate it without ever totally eliminating it. In fact, the required decontamination conditions are so intense that many surgeons don't meet them for fear of damaging the tools themselves.

Of course, the patients in Collinge's study didn't have Alzheimer's.

They may never have got it. So Collinge considered other possibilities. Maybe CJD somehow made the patients' brains more vulnerable to Alzheimer's. Maybe the CJD prions seeded the growth of beta-amyloid; prions can do this by a mysterious process dubbed cross-seeding. But in every other CJD case Collinge's team examined, none had comparable levels of beta-amyloid. Plus, both seeds were found physically far apart, which was hardly convincing evidence for one corrupting the other.

When word of Collinge's discovery got out, people started worrying they might catch Alzheimer's after seeing their dentist. CAN GOING TO THE DENTIST GIVE YOU ALZHEIMER'S? proposed the UK's *Daily Mail* newspaper. Fortunately, that scenario seems far-fetched, and this small, inconclusive study certainly shouldn't make you cancel your next dental check-up or hospital appointment.[8]

Nevertheless, until the human source of these patients' amyloid is confirmed, similar transmission events can't be ruled out. So in a desperate bid to learn more, Collinge and others are still searching for the original growth hormone extracts, prepared decades ago at various locations. If found, all they need to do to prove human transmission is follow Mathias Jucker's lead, i.e. inject an animal with it and then see if it develops Alzheimer's pathology. From this strange coupling emerged an inescapable question. Alzheimer's could be spontaneous. It could be genetic. Could it also be acquired?

John Collinge, seated in his office at the National Prion Clinic in London, his desk covered with issues of *Nature* and government reports, told me that he doesn't want to scare anyone. Alzheimer's is *not* contagious, he assured me. But – and there is undoubtedly a 'but' – it may be transmissible under certain circumstances. 'Prions are lethal pathogens,' he said in a quiet, measured tone, 'and I don't think that beta-amyloid is a lethal pathogen that passes from person to person in the same way. But the idea that amyloid seeds is not speculative. It seeds by definition.'

Collinge is a mild-mannered man with deep-set eyes, bushy eyebrows, and a stratospheric intellect. He's been studying prions for more than thirty years. He was one of the early investigators showing that they're transmissible. When the UK's bovine spongiform encephalopathy (BSE, or 'mad cow') epidemic manifested in humans as CJD – so-called variant-CJD – in the 1990s, the government appointed him as their go-to guy to defuse a potential prion time bomb and thwart another epidemic. And it really was a time bomb: scientists had discovered that prions could incubate in humans for decades without producing any symptoms – providing yet another ominous unknown. Funded by the Department of Health, Collinge set up a National Prion Clinic in 1998 and used patient post-mortems to amass a natural history of the pathogens.

Although CJD was his primary focus, he was acutely aware of the implications for other neurological disorders, and always saw Alzheimer's as 'part of the mission'. The conspicuous features of rare diseases, he knew, give clues to common diseases. 'That's the way I've always seen prion diseases,' he said. 'If proteins can do this, it isn't just going to be about CJD; it's going to open the door to so many things, and at the top of that list is Alzheimer's.'

One of the first things the UK government wanted Collinge to do was investigate better ways to sterilise surgical tools. Politicians were slowly catching up with what scientists were seeing and were understandably worried about the risk of hospital-acquired infection, given how seemingly indestructible prions are. So they invested more than £10 million in Collinge and other researchers to devise a potent decontamination technology. Seven years, 400 combinations of detergents and enzymes later, Collinge had done just that. He'd made a biological washing powder that eliminated prions from metal by a million-fold, below all limits of detection. The technology was commercialised by the American chemical company DuPont, a cheap disinfectant product called RelyOn™ was manufactured, and a UK scientific advisory committee recommended that the government use it.

Blood transfusion was the next big concern. Without any blood test for prions, it was impossible to know how they were circulating in the population. It was an invisible mystery, with a bad track record: in the 1980s and 1990s, UK blood transfusions led to over 4,000 haemophiliacs contracting hepatitis C and 1,200 infections of HIV, resulting in over 2,000 deaths. Since prions can lurk in the body for decades before any symptoms emerge, a good blood test was even more urgent. And so Collinge delivered yet again. In February 2011, by exploiting the prions' affinity for metal, he invented an ingenious test that uses metal powder to detect prions in the blood. With a sensitivity of one part per 10 billion, it was 100,000 times more sensitive than every other method. Again, a panel of experts recommended the government use it.

It had been hard, expensive, but we'd got ahead of this one. The mistakes of the past weren't going to be repeated. Reason and prudence and science had prevailed.

But astonishingly, the British government chose to use neither the disinfectant nor the blood test. When it came to using the disinfectant in a hospital setting, they put up so much red tape that DuPont was only allowed to conduct one trial (which was a success). Then the same advisory committee that recommended the disinfectant told DuPont that the British National Health Service simply wouldn't use it; after all, who would bother with an additional sterilisation step when the prion prevalence in the population was still unknown? As for the blood test, when Collinge sought to try it on 20,000 UK and 20,000 US blood samples – for £750,000 – the government rejected the proposal. At a House of Commons Science and Technology Committee session in 2014, Sally Davies, the government's Chief Medical Officer, said that 'the government had limited budgets for healthcare, public health and research,' adding that it had already 'given a lot of money to this area of prion research, particularly to Professor Collinge'.

Collinge was flabbergasted. The government had spent more than £10 million specifically to develop technologies to detect and decontaminate prions, deadly pathogens that were so resilient they made viruses and bacteria look pathetic, and then ditched the entire enterprise as soon as it succeeded.

Fellow experts were similarly nonplussed. Many gave testimony at the House of Commons session in support of Collinge. The blood test was 'the next logical step' said Marc Turner, director of the Scottish National Blood Transfusion Services. There was 'a great deal of scope' for these methods, echoed Roland Salmon, chair of the UK's Advisory Committee on Dangerous Pathogens. Obviously, the next move 'would be to conduct a study of the UK population using blood samples to understand what the frequency of prion infection in the blood actually is', insisted Lorna Williamson, Research Director at the NHS Blood and Transfusion group.

The report documenting this is a galling read.[9] The Science and Technology Committee said the government's behaviour was 'unacceptable', concluding: 'We simply do not know, at present, how many people have been exposed to prions and what the implications of this might be . . . There is an urgent need to reduce this uncertainty.'

Then Collinge's Alzheimer's paper came out. Wanting to avoid a public health scare, Collinge told the Department of Health about his findings before they were published. Again, he expressed his concern about the prion threat, and pointed out that many experts did indeed think that the eight CJD patients would have eventually got Alzheimer's. This really wasn't just about CJD any more.

Instead of revisiting the issue, however, the same Chief Medical Officer set out to deride Collinge's study. In a bizarre perversion of conduct, Davies took it upon herself to break the terms of *Nature*'s embargo and tell Richard Horton, editor of rival journal the *Lancet*, about the study. She asked Horton how he could help downplay the results. So the *Lancet* published an editorial slamming Collinge's data.[10] It was a strange move, seeing as *Nature* had already vetted the paper by peer review and Collinge had explained the study's caveats. Then, Davies told the press: 'I can assure people that the NHS has extremely stringent procedures in place to minimise infection risk from surgical equipment, and patients are very well protected.'[11] Formally true, of course – just not when it came to prions.

The *Lancet*'s main gripe was that the study hadn't proven human transmission definitively, a critique Collinge vehemently contests. 'Our paper doesn't *prove* that it's been transmitted this way,' he explained. 'It's very hard to prove anything in biology, as you know. It's rather like the arguments twenty years ago that asked, "Can you prove variant-CJD is caused by BSE?" Well, no one's going to inject children with BSE and see whether they get CJD, but that's how you would prove it. So it's always going to be a collection of evidence. And you reach a point where it just seems so clear, and the weight of all this literature suggests that protein seeding is clearly an aspect of what's going on in Alzheimer's.'

Although the headlines weren't great – the *Daily Mirror*: YOU CAN CATCH ALZHEIMER'S; the *Independent*: ALZHEIMER'S MAY BE A TRANSMISSIBLE INFECTION – the articles themselves were good. Collinge had spent hours explaining his data to the press, and was pretty satisfied with the coverage. The *Lancet*'s editorial took more issue with his choice of words than the media's. He had called the discovery a 'paradigm shift', when, according to them, it was 'a long way from a true "paradigm shift"'.

So was Kuhn's accolade justified? 'It's a completely different way of thinking about a disease,' Collinge emphasised. 'We used to think of Alzheimer's as this spontaneous, mysterious process that may be caused by genetic changes. But now, thinking of it as these protein seeds forming and spreading in the brain, which in certain circumstances can actually be transmitted by medical accidents . . .' He paused and raised his eyebrows at me. 'That's a shift in thinking for most people.'

Despite my ingrained scepticism, I found myself agreeing with him.

The implications of the prion paradigm are far-reaching. A 'transmissibility hypothesis' of Alzheimer's is forcing hospitals around the world to engage in an uncomfortable degree of self-scrutiny, and some have already begun to do so: scientists at the Center for Disease Control and Prevention (CDC) in Atlanta, Georgia, are now helping pathologists trawl through archives of post-mortem brain tissue to check for signs of amyloid seeds; the Pitié-Salpêtrière Hospital in Paris, France, is doing the same, as are several groups in Austria, Switzerland and Japan. While the evidence remains circumstantial – indeed, in March 2016 Pierluigi Nicotera of the German Centre for Neurodegenerative Diseases in Bonn told *Nature*'s Alison Abbott: 'We have to remember that there is no conclusive evidence that seeds of amyloid can transmit actual disease or that amyloid spreads in the brain in a prion-like way' – others are not so sceptical. 'In my opinion, all amyloids should be considered dangerous until proven safe,' said Adriano Aguzzi of the University Hospital Zurich in Switzerland.[12] I lean more towards the latter viewpoint by virtue of the oft-cited reasoning of astronomer Carl Sagan: absence of evidence is not evidence of absence. It will of course be years before we know the true extent of the role prions play in Alzheimer's, but dismissing a disturbing hypothesis does nothing to help patients or the public appreciate the complexity of this seemingly ordinary disease. And by the mid-twenty-first century, when the need for treatment turns from necessity to urgency, we will need to have crossed every possibility off our list.

17

Looking but not Seeing

I felt totally alone, with the world receding away from me in every direction, and you could have used my anger to weld steel.

Sir Terry Pratchett, Alzheimer's Society, 2008

THE DRIVE UP to Liverpool was becoming second nature to Pam and Richard Faulkner. From their rural home in south-western England, the route followed the M5 towards Birmingham, past the rolling hills of the Peak District, and on through Cheshire, before finally ending up in the hometown of Richard's parents. It only took about two and a half hours. But during one such trip, on a January day in 2013, the couple found themselves approaching heavy traffic.

Thinking on her feet, Pam pulled out a map. She'd learned how to navigate when she was a child, and often took on the role of map-reader during family excursions. They weren't far from Liverpool. This would be a doddle, she thought.

Staring at the map, however, she couldn't quite believe what she was seeing. Or rather, what she *wasn't* seeing. Everything looked muddled: the roads, the junctions, the symbols – none of it made any sense. She closed her eyes and then looked again . . . it was the same: completely unintelligible. Richard couldn't understand what the problem was. Pam was only fifty-nine, hardly the age to be having such an odd mental lapse. But this wasn't an everyday slip-up, Pam realised. It was something else. It was as if, in the blink of an eye, she'd forgotten how to read English.

Flummoxed, Pam's first recourse was to get new glasses (while Richard looked into buying a satnav). Though Pam had recently given up night driving – after the headlights from oncoming traffic frequently made her see a dizzying blue after-image – her optician couldn't find anything particularly wrong with her sight. And so, at a loss, she simply put the incident behind her and went back to enjoying early retirement.

A few months later, the problem returned. This time it was jigsaw puzzles and reading. Thousand-piece puzzles were Pam's passion; anything less she deemed 'wimpy'. But while deftly assembling her latest puzzle – an exotic Spanish garden – she suddenly noticed that she could no longer join the pieces together. The order was right; she just couldn't physically align each piece. Similarly, news-paper columns became impossible to follow unless the text was justified on both sides. If not, she would reach the end of a line and then simply not know where to go next. And then, in June 2014, Pam found herself on the bathroom floor with no memory of how she got there. She'd had a seizure.

At first the neurologists struggled to provide an answer. Nearly all other aspects of Pam's cognitive faculties were normal, as was an MRI of her brain. They diagnosed epilepsy but couldn't explain why the seizures had started. Unsure exactly what they were dealing with, the neurologists prescribed anti-epileptic medication while a GP referred Pam to a memory clinic.

But in a battery of memory tests Pam did surprisingly well. So the doctor pulled out a test she hadn't performed since she was trained. It was a neuropsychological test of visual perception, depicting various objects at strange angles which are then rotated until the subject can accurately identify them. On this test, Pam was 'bloody awful', as she put it. On 15 July 2015 Pam finally got her true diagnosis. It was Alzheimer's – but not as we know it.

Visual Alzheimer's, otherwise known as Posterior Cortical Atrophy (PCA), was first described in 1988 by the American neurologist Frank Benson.[1] Unlike typical Alzheimer's, people with PCA retain their memories, thinking skills and personal insight until much later in the disease. A patient with PCA, Benson wrote, is 'aware of current events, and [shows] considerable insight into his or her predicament'. Instead, they experience a profound and surreal visual dementia. In addition to hallucinations, there are reports of people suddenly losing the ability to read, to accurately perceive movement and the size of objects, to recognise faces and find their way around familiar environments. There's even a case of an individual who began seeing the world upside-down, in complete 180-degree reverse.

The English fantasy novelist Terry Pratchett had this kind of Alzheimer's, which he wryly called his 'embuggerance'. In December 2007, upon learning his fate, Pratchett launched a relentless, seven-year campaign to put PCA in the public eye. Having published more than seventy books in a career spanning almost fifty years, he was furious that such an illness could strip the mind – and indeed the mind's eye – so effortlessly. 'I have the opposite of a superpower,' he later wrote with trademark good humour. 'Sometimes I cannot see what is there. I see the teacup with my eyes, but my brain refuses to send me the teacup message. It's very Zen. First there is no teacup and then, because I know there is a teacup, the teacup will appear the next time I look.'[2] Happily adopting the nickname 'Mr Alzheimer's', Pratchett gave hundreds of interviews and made an award-winning documentary about his plight called *Living with Alzheimer's*.

It worked, too; nearly everyone I met for this book mentioned his name. During his final years, Pratchett travelled the globe in search of a cure, and was not averse to trying experimental therapies, including an 'anti-dementia helmet' – thought, though certainly not proven, to treat Alzheimer's by firing a burst of light into the skull to stimulate the growth of new brain cells. In 2014, one year before his death, he published a short volume titled *Shaking Hands with Death*, lucidly relating the feeling of PCA:

> Imagine that you're in a very, very slow motion car crash. Nothing much seems to be happening. There's an occasional little bang, a crunch, a screw pops out and spins across the dashboard as if we're

in Apollo 13. But the radio is still playing, the heater is on and it doesn't seem all that bad, except for the certain knowledge that sooner or later you will be definitely going head first through the windscreen.

That's just one example. In his book *The Mind's Eye*, neurologist Oliver Sacks described an instance of PCA in a pianist named Lilian Kallir, who could no longer read music and, when confronted by people's faces, said, 'It is not a blur, it's a mush.' So peculiar was her affliction that, in the months following their meeting, the pair became locked in a cat-and-mouse game for answers, with Sacks repeatedly showing her different pictures and shapes to elucidate the cause, and Lilian constantly thwarting his efforts with her baffling responses.[3] He studied her in the familiar surroundings of her apartment in Manhattan, New York, where she organised her belongings based on size and shape, instead of meaning – like 'an illiterate person might arrange the books in a library', Sacks noted. Accompanying her on a trip to the supermarket, he noticed that her success was predicated on memorising the different blends of colour forming each aisle: colour, he said, was 'her most immediately visible cue, recognisable when nothing else is'.

Due to its strikingly diverse symptoms, PCA is thought to have gone undetected for decades, perhaps centuries. It's still not known how many people have it, but some estimates put it at 5–10 per cent of all early-onset Alzheimer's cases.[4] To be clear, PCA isn't a symptom of Alzheimer's: it's a different *form* of Alzheimer's altogether. Many patients, including Pam, end up having unnecessary eye operations such as cataract surgery. Others, it's thought, are simply never diagnosed. But there is nothing wrong with these people's eyes. As an organ the eye only detects light from the outside world: after focusing on the retina, light is absorbed by a layer of photoreceptor cells and then sent inside the brain as electrical signals via the optic nerve. Vision itself is crafted deep within the circuitry of the brain.

Look around you. Wherever you are, every aspect of the image you're seeing – the assorted shapes, sizes, colours, depths, orientations and motions – are all generated by different networks of neurons in your brain. The seamless and movie-like projection we actually experience is a total illusion. Our world isn't really 'out there' in the way we imagine; it's compartmentalised internally, and then stitched together into a neuronal mosaic situated at the back of the brain, known as the visual cortex. Take me: I'm presently sitting in a departure lounge at Heathrow Airport. If just one part of my brain's visual cortex shuts down, the people walking past me might suddenly appear to move in snapshots. If another fails, I wouldn't know how wide to open my hands to grasp my cup of coffee.

So it's no surprise that plaques and tangles in the visual cortex spell disaster. And that's exactly what happens in PCA. The pathology of Alzheimer's starts there, and then spreads, years later, to the brain's memory centres – the hippocampus and cortex. The cause is even more mysterious than classic Alzheimer's. No genetic mutations have been confirmed, and the idea that APOE4 is somehow involved is heavily disputed. It eventually shrinks the brain in much the same way as Alzheimer's. Patients are given the standard Alzheimer's drug – an acetylcholinesterase inhibitor – because neurologists simply don't know what else to do.

But the riddle of PCA, I was about to learn, is beginning to unfold. And under close interrogation, it has some interesting things to say about typical Alzheimer's.

One of the researchers at the forefront of PCA is Sebastian Crutch at University College London. Convinced that visual Alzheimer's holds important societal messages as well as biological intrigues, he decided to investigate using methods as unconventional as the illness itself. 'It really is the same disease,' Crutch said to me over the clatter of tourists when I met him for coffee at the London Science Museum. 'It's just in a different place.'

Crutch hadn't chosen to meet at the Science Museum on a nerdy impulse. He was here to tell the public about a project called 'Seeing What They See', a highly innovative attempt to enter the minds, so to speak, of PCA sufferers by building specific environments and then using motion-tracking sensors to see how they navigate. 'The idea is that we can support their behaviour if we're aware of what helps and what doesn't,' explained Crutch. 'For example, we used some empty rooms – normal rooms: beige walls, wooden floors, lighting overhead – and measured how long it took for them to walk through one of three target doors which are illuminated by a moving cube. We've done experiments guiding them down corridors using different shapes, because Alzheimer's isn't just about disabilities; it's about capabilities as well. And if we can understand what aspects of people's vision *are* still functioning, we can use that sort of information.'

According to Crutch, there's a reason people with PCA preserve their memory for so long. On the one hand, he explained, there's good evidence that genetic variants in the visual cortex cause Alzheimer's to ransack this region first. But one can also argue that these genes are actually protecting the brain's memory centres by channelling the disease elsewhere, effectively cordoning memory off. That's the viewpoint Crutch stands by. 'If there's something in PCA that actually protects your memory, something which means the disease isn't pushing into the hippocampus to the same extent as in typical Alzheimer's, I want to know about that.'

Thirty-eight years old, with sleek dark hair and pale green eyes, Crutch comes from a family of engineers. His grandmother had Alzheimer's, although his desire to do something about it appeared long before her mind fell. Throughout our conversation he animated every point with quick hand gestures and an intense stare. So eager was he to help me, in fact, he emailed me a study his team have yet to publish. It's a rare delight to see the final draft of another group's work before publication; many researchers are not so trusting. But the impression I got from Crutch was that he deemed this area of research too important to play politics.

The study involved a crack team of forty-four scientists from seven different countries. They'd genotyped some 300 PCA patients and identified a host of new genetic risk factors. One of them, a gene dubbed SEMA3C, appears to corroborate Crutch's hypothesis of memory-shielding genes in Alzheimer's. In the visual cortex, SEMA3C aids the development of vision; but in the hippocampus, it supports learning and memory. It can do both because it's thought to control 'functional network connectivity' – that is, how the brain is wired to generate different cognitive processes. So when Alzheimer's strikes, something about SEMA3C's wide-ranging abilities might safeguard memory by redirecting the disease to the visual cortex. If Crutch can figure out what that ability is, he could theoretically design a drug that directs Alzheimer's away from the hippocampus, and every other region of sacrosanct cognition, to some other place. Ideally, that place would be the brain's glymphatic pathway, the system of glial cells and spinal fluid we saw in chapter thirteen, which clears the brain of waste products and is thought to underlie how the brain cleans itself during sleep. In this scenario, plaques and tangles would be the waste products, leaving improved cognition in their wake.

PCA has thus revealed a weak link in the chain of Alzheimer's, in that plaques and tangles may be far more mobile, and in turn more directable, than ever imagined.

'All I could think was, how do we move forward?' Pam said while I rested the Dictaphone on her living room table. It was a wet January afternoon in 2016 and I was talking to Pam and Richard at their English countryside home in a pint-sized village in Gloucestershire. 'Because I didn't want to cry, or hide in a corner and shake like a jelly. I just wanted to keep moving.'

Pam is a bright, tech-savvy woman who grew up in South Yorkshire. As an only child, her parents doted on her – especially her father, a blasting engineer. So while the local norm in the 1970s was for young girls to find a suitable husband and stay at home, Pam decided to study physics at Oxford University instead. Working in the then burgeoning computer industry, she met Richard, a like-minded computer whizz whom she felt was more than suitable. The pair never had children, and have spent their days travelling, devouring books, enjoying the company of friends, and savouring English sunsets.

'At the moment, it's sort of okay,' she explained with some hesitance. 'I'm taking Aricept, which is definitely making me feel less fuzzy.' As I continued to scribble everything the Dictaphone could not capture, I noticed that Richard made a point of giving Pam a white mug for her tea: the colour contrast is now a necessity. Bright or shiny objects don't register with her, he explained. Even a teaspoon placed against their dark kitchen worktop may not be seen.

Richard recalled one incident when they went trekking in Cornwall. It was a sunny day and the couple were traversing a coastal path that would take them down to the beach below when, suddenly, Pam froze. She could no longer see the path in front of her. The sunlight twinkling on the ocean had completely paralysed her gaze. 'It was as if she couldn't get her brain to move her eyes on to the path,' said Richard, 'so she grabbed my hand and we gently walked down together. That's our normal practice now.'

But the most tormenting loss for Pam is no longer being able to read. The proud owner of a library containing some 3,000 books, she's not ready to convert to audiobooks. To demonstrate, she asked Richard to hand her a magazine and invited me to sit next to her. She began reading one of the columns aloud, but quickly stopped at the end of the first line.

'Where do I go next?' she asked me.

I pointed to the line below.

'Okay,' she acknowledged, 'but where's the next line?'

'This *is* the next line,' I said.

She sighed in exasperation. Despite seeing the same thing as I was, her brain refused to comprehend it.

'But now it's everything,' she confessed. 'I can't pour drinks into glasses any more. I can't chop an onion or do up shoelaces, because I can't line anything up. In the garden I'd cut my fingers instead of the stems.

'Pressure is also becoming a problem. I struggle with zips now because I don't know how hard to pull. When I cut into food with a knife, I don't know how hard to press.

'What about soup?' I asked.

'No, eating soup I can't do. Think about it: you have to take the spoon, pick some soup up in the spoon, hold it flat, and then get it into your mouth without pouring it down yourself. But I don't know what's flat.'

A healthy brain performs these everyday tasks by activating a region called the posterior parietal cortex (PPC). This area is vital for planned movement and our apprehension of shapes. Activity in the PPC increases when subjects are asked to virtually navigate a familiar environment.[5] The PPC is also thought to influence eye movements and how we grasp the location of objects in space.[6] In Pam's brain these functions are essentially scrambled because plaques and tangles disrupt the way electrical signals travel between nerve cells. As the functions of her PPC continue to fail, Pam's symptoms will manifest in ever more strange and unexpected ways. (One patient Pam met can recognise her left and right shoe, but has no idea whether they are the same style and colour as each other.)

Like Terry Pratchett, Richard and Pam decided to tell everyone about their baffling predicament. Richard made flyers titled WHAT'S GOT INTO PAM? and took them door-to-door. Under the subtitle WHAT CAN YOU DO? he wrote: 'Treat Pam as you always have, but have patience with her when she is finding her way around and understand when her memory fails her.' Like so many Alzheimer's sufferers, Pam wants awareness, not sympathy; action, not sorrow. She and Richard regularly attend PCA support meetings and help out with Crutch's 'Seeing What They See' project.

It feels uncomfortable to say, but one of the benefits of this kind of Alzheimer's is that the person retains a certain degree of insight. Pam's world is slowly collapsing around her. She knows that what she's experiencing is only a preview of what's to come; that her memory will be next; that there will come a point when she can no longer find the bathroom in her own home. And yet, for the time being, she's able to comment on her plight in a way most others cannot. Her Alzheimer's can still 'fit into a logical world', as she elegantly put it, adding that 'the wanting to know, to understand what's happening, is still there.'

People often mistakenly presume that there is one face to Alzheimer's, but Pam has shown there is another. She's a reminder of our endless duty to define and redefine Alzheimer's, and a reminder that people's experience of it is something no brain scan or blood test can ever communicate.

18

Between the Devil and the Deep Blue Sea

> The most fruitful basis for the discovery of a new drug is to start with an old drug.
>
> Sir James Black

SIX HOURS WAS all it took. In a burst of potency and precision the drug found its target, locking on to receptors deep within the brain to jumpstart a molecular cascade. Like a pinball obeying the laws of motion, the impact ricocheted through neurons, reordering their inner 'cogs' and 'springs' until a new set of genes sprang into action. The mouse woke to the now familiar feelings of confusion and forgetfulness. But it felt better somehow – smarter. Of course, it would never know that a drug had just eviscerated a quarter of the amyloid in its plaque-riddled brain. Nor was it aware, three days later, that half of the amyloid would vanish. All it knew was that it had finally remembered how to ruffle tissue paper into a satisfying nest.

The scientist watching couldn't believe her luck, for this drug was already approved in humans. For the past thirteen years it had been used not for Alzheimer's, but for skin cancer.

In 2010, as the Alzheimer's vaccination yielded unexpected insights, other researchers decided to do a little lateral thinking of their own. Among them were the American neuroscientist Tom Curran and the French biologist Yves Christen, who convened a meeting on 26 April in Paris. The topic under discussion was a remarkable tale of yin and yang: how Alzheimer's and cancer are actually two sides of the same coin. The audience, having just started to dissect the biology of dementia, suddenly found themselves squaring an unexpected circle. How can cancer, the uncontrolled growth and proliferation of a single cell, be at all related to a disease characterised by countless cells simply withering away and dying?

There was, no doubt, a connection. Statistics had shown that people who get Alzheimer's have a lower risk of developing cancer.[1] Inversely, if you develop cancer you're less likely to get Alzheimer's. The same holds true for cancer and Parkinson's, and cancer and motor neuron disease. Genetic observations also spotlighted a link, in that cancer-affiliated genes − like p53 (mutated in half of all human cancers), ATM, CDK5, mTOR and PTEN (acronyms hauntingly familiar to many cancer victims) − all appeared to overlap with cellular pathways underlying Alzheimer's.[2] It was as if a pendulum was swinging between the two. Perhaps, then, slowing the arc towards one could slow the arc towards the other.

From 8.30 a.m. to the close of the day, more than a dozen speakers tried to build a case for how this might be possible. Cancer is known to be an aberration of the cell's normal life and death mechanisms: mutated genes derail the cell cycle and lethal replication is the consequence. But neurons don't divide, and so instead of impacting the cell cycle, neuronal damage appears to activate proteins that converge on the 'death pathway': a network of tightly controlled proteins that carefully dismantle the neuron from within. And this is where things get interesting, for many of those proteins are also involved in cancer. Maybe hitting Alzheimer's with cancer drugs − drugs that work by essentially meddling with these protein networks − was therefore worth a shot. Maybe, as one French journalist wrote at the time, 'this cross-fertilisation between the fields may well go on to bear a wonderful new crop'.[3]

The first to reap such a harvest was neither a cancer biologist nor a qualified neuroscientist. A spunky twenty-two-year-old graduate student at Case Western Reserve University, in Cleveland, Ohio,

Paige Cramer was a novice in the eyes of her mentors. And yet, on 23 March 2012, she submitted evidence to the pages of *Science*, arguably the most prestigious scientific journal, that a thirteen-year-old skin cancer drug called bexarotene could completely reverse the symptoms of Alzheimer's in a matter of days.[4] This was in mice, of course, not humans. But the effects were so profound that such a detail had – for once – taken a back seat.

Originally from the emerald-green coast of Pensacola, Florida, Cramer grew up in a studious household. Her father is a physician and scientist, her mother an attorney in healthcare law. She told me that she remembers many evenings spent around the dinner table discussing diseases and puzzling scientific problems. She was almost custom-built for biomedical science, I thought. The scales were tipped during Cramer's freshman year of college, when her best friend became paraplegic after a spinal cord injury, and Cramer decided that neurology needed more detectives.

Brand-named Targretin®, bexarotene was designed to treat T-cell lymphoma – a rare type of skin cancer caused by white blood cells called T-cell lymphocytes – but it wasn't very effective. Oncologists only prescribed it when patients didn't respond to better medications. 'Truth be told, I'd never heard of it,' Cramer's supervisor, Gary Landreth, told me. 'It's still controversial in the cancer business, because no one really knows how it's supposed to work in T-cell lymphoma.' So how was a cancer drug supposed to work in Alzheimer's? I wondered.

I kept digging. It turned out that what enticed Cramer was the drug's ability to strike at the innermost chords of neuronal chemistry. Inside every cell, genes are activated by a special class of proteins called transcription factors. These proteins physically bind to DNA and then race along its threads like bows on a string. The result is a close copy of the gene, called RNA, which then rises up to ultimately do its job in the form of a protein. By boosting the activity of a transcription factor called RXR (retinoid X receptor) bexarotene thus acts as a kind of DNA conductor, directing the cell to prioritise certain 'notes', or proteins, over others.

But Cramer's attraction to RXR was something more than mere chemistry. Once active, RXR appears to control the levels of apolipoprotein E (APOE), the same molecule that won Allen Roses both fame and exile in the 1990s. Now here was a link worth exploring, Cramer thought. In the twenty years since Roses had pinpointed APOE4 as the prime genetic risk for Alzheimer's, attitudes towards it remained mixed, and the trials targeting it had all run aground.

But if one could truly modify APOE4, half of all Alzheimer's cases might be history. And the upshot didn't end there: good evidence suggests that APOE proteins help clear the brain of beta-amyloid. The details are typically fuzzy; for instance, it isn't known whether APOE does this by physically latching on to beta-amyloid (like a Venus flytrap), or if it somehow recycles the plaques by other means. But in any event, the prospect of a tool capable of targeting two of the three main disease culprits was irresistible.

And so, in an act as routine as it was startling, Cramer convinced a physician in her department to write her a prescription, and then wandered down to her local pharmacy to pick up the would-be Alzheimer's cure. 'It's not really legal to do that,' Cramer said to me over the phone, 'but I was just a naive graduate student, one that was willing to try anything.'

Upon returning to the lab, Cramer broke the cancer pills apart and began feeding them to her mice. Several hours later, the mice's beta-amyloid levels dropped by 25 per cent. Within 72 hours the drop hit 50 per cent, an unprecedented result. She witnessed this in transgenic mice harbouring both Carol Jennings's and Victoria Huntley's genetic mutations, as well as mice engineered to display a particularly rapid and aggressive form of Alzheimer's.

By meticulously observing the mice's behaviour over the next three days, Cramer also discovered that they were nesting just like they used to. Lab mice are usually given pieces of pressed cotton which they chew up and shred into nests. Transgenic Alzheimer's mice lose the ability to do this, kind of like how human Alzheimer's patients lose the ability to dress themselves, but Cramer's mice were suddenly able to resume their nest-making.

The mice that had been fed bexarotene also far exceeded their sick counterparts in maze trials and other tests of memory. One such test is known as contextual fear conditioning, in which a mouse receives a stimulus (usually a loud noise) followed by an unpleasant sensation (usually a mild foot shock), forcing it to adopt the stereotypical behavioural response of freezing like a statue. It's somewhat cruel, I concede, but it's highly informative. Of all the emotions, fear is perhaps the most closely connected to memory. Everyone remembers frightening experiences. It's also an evolutionary imperative, and so organisms quickly learn what to be fearful of and respond in the same way at the mere sight of it. This was most disturbingly demonstrated in 1920 using a human child. 'The Little Albert Experiment', conducted by US psychologists John Watson and Rosalie Rayner, trained a nine-month-old baby to associate loud banging noises with the sight of a white rat. Thereafter, Albert became petrified when confronted by anything resembling a white rat – a white dog, a white coat, the white beard of a Santa Claus mask. The memory was seared indelibly on his mind.

In the brain, fear conditioning is governed by an ancient interplay between the hippocampus and a neighbouring region called the amygdala. For Cramer, this gave the perfect opportunity to see how deep bexarotene's effects on memory really went, because a good fear response is predicated on a healthy hippocampus. 'Think about the idea as you hear a train,' she explained. 'Generally speaking, if you're near a train track you'll look both ways, because you have that association of *moving-train-equals-danger; be careful*. Someone whose memory hasn't developed properly, or whose memory is impaired, won't make that connection and will continue to walk near a track without looking.' That Cramer's demented mice could again be fear conditioned, therefore, indicated a powerful resurgence in neuronal connectivity.

That wasn't all. In considering how else she could assess their memory, Cramer decided to focus on smell. It may surprise you to learn that one of the first things many Alzheimer's patients experience is 'anosmia', the partial or near total loss of smell. What shouldn't surprise you is that memory and smell are intimately linked. I for one, at the faintest whiff of a familiar scent, am instantly flooded with images and feelings of past events; even memories I'd long forgotten come crashing back. It's due to the way smell is wired in the brain, being processed by a region called the olfactory bulb. And like the amygdala, the olfactory bulb sits right next to the hippocampus.

Interestingly, Alzheimer's patients appear to have an especially hard time smelling peanut butter. A 2013 study performed by Jennifer Stamps, a researcher in the Department of Food Science and Human Nutrition at the University of Florida, instructed a group of patients to close their eyes and identify the smell from a container holding 14 grams (a tablespoon) of the condiment.[5] When the patients struggled to detect the scent, Stamps moved the container 1 centimetre closer to their nostrils. She found that Alzheimer's patients required the peanut butter to be about 10 centimetres closer than both healthy people and patients with other types of dementia. The anosmia was largely confined to the left nostril, which is thought to be because Alzheimer's damages the left side of the brain more than the right. The relationship between smell and Alzheimer's is now so well documented that scientists are trying to use smell as a biomarker for early diagnosis.

By measuring the electrical activity of a circuit within the olfactory bulb, known as the piriform cortex (from the Latin *pyriformis*, meaning 'pear-shaped'), Cramer found that her transgenic animals' sense of smell was being enhanced by drug treatment. 'This is really exciting,' she noted, with audible exhilaration, 'because it's another benefit for neuronal networks, for the strengthening of connections between brain regions.'

Landreth echoed her excitement. 'In mice it's like magic. The effect of this drug is so rapid in reversing the pathology. Think about this: bexarotene is the first example of a drug that actually modifies Alzheimer's disease mechanisms. And it works in thirty days.'

I myself remember the buzz surrounding this discovery. I penned a piece for *Pi*, University College London's student newspaper, calling attention to it (much to my supervisor's chagrin; I could have been doing more experiments instead). Listening to Cramer and Landreth retell the story, something about it still stirred me. It all started with a doctor handing her a prescription and telling her to head to a drug store. Was the elusive cure for Alzheimer's sitting on a shelf in our pharmacies all along?

I wasn't alone in that wish. Cramer's findings drew instant attention from the press. Landreth received a torrent of correspondence from reporters and, more importantly, the relatives of Alzheimer's patients themselves. 'We published in February,' he stated, 'and I was not able to answer my phone until November. I got hundreds of calls and emails from all these desperate people. My secretary was in tears listening to their stories. It was heartbreaking.'

'People want something,' Cramer elaborated. 'They *need* something.' Despite warnings about using the drug off-label, some people went ahead anyway, more than willing to take matters into their own hands. In the press the story of one Mandy Vear, from Rossendale, England, began to surface.[6] As Vear's father's condition was descending into outright violence against his family, she pleaded with her doctor to write him a prescription for bexarotene. But the physician refused, for bexarotene's side effects cast a dark shadow by raising triglycerides: blood fats linked to diabetes and heart disease.

Another story featured an anonymous Belgian patient whose physician agreed. Sixty-eight years old, the man reportedly took the drug every day for twenty-three months and was monitored by a team at the Université catholique de Louvain, in Brussels, Belgium.[7] Tantalisingly, his memory somewhat improved and he scored higher in several tests of cognition. The problem, as one would expect, is that there was no way to rule out a placebo effect. And so this anecdotal case fossilised as just that: anecdotal, informal, unreliable. 'You've just got to take it for what it's worth,' Landreth made clear to me. 'It supports the idea, but you certainly wouldn't base any subsequent action on a case report.'

But where were the human trials? I wondered.

I learned that four other groups, inspired by Cramer's discovery, had already set about replicating her data. Before any discovery is given credit, before it can launch human trials, it faces the gauntlet of widespread replication and doubt. This isn't pretty; scientists can shoot down someone's work with the accuracy of an Olympic archer. Which, unfortunately, is exactly what they did. Just as Cramer and Landreth were pushing for clinical trials, all four groups announced that they categorically could not reproduce Cramer's data. Had she made a mistake? Could her discovery be an illusion, a quirk of her batch of mice, perhaps? Was this all just a tempest in a teapot?

In May 2013 *Nature* published a disheartening article outlining the dissenters' views.[8] Their chief criticism was that bexarotene didn't actually affect Alzheimer's plaques. Rather, the drug diminished levels of a smaller, free-floating form of beta-amyloid called oligo-meric amyloid: a kind of intermediate brand of the toxin, which clusters together long before plaques appear. Yet many believed this type of amyloid was more central to the disease process. A stack of scientific literature had shown that oligomeric amyloid could scramble synaptic communication like hail bombarding a television antenna. And while plaques certainly looked more deadly, their invisible predecessors correlated better with memory impairment and cognitive decline. Some even claimed that clinical trials had failed because they'd tried to remove plaques, when they should really have tried to remove oligomers.

For Landreth, it was all a lot of hot air. 'It pissed me off that this entire discussion centred on plaques, when we explicitly showed that plaques don't matter! All the plaques say is "things have gone badly in the brain". But if improved memory and cognition is the ultimate goal, why should plaques matter? It's clear that these small oligomeric species affect synapses, and I think we improved the animals' behaviour by removing them from the brain.'

He was also quick to point out that other groups had prepared the drug differently. They'd dissolved its raw powder in an artificial liquid, instead of simply using the pill form, as Cramer had. The reason that matters, Landreth maintained, is that the former stays in the blood for minutes while the latter remains in circulation for hours. And in the realm of molecular genetics, that disparity was titanic.

Although Landreth's rejoinder wasn't enough for Big Pharma to weigh in, others weren't ready to see the lead so easily dispatched. A group of private donors – all anonymous Alzheimer's relatives – raised over $1 million to fund a small clinical trial, led by Jeffrey Cummings at the Lou Ruvo Center for Brain Health in Las Vegas, Nevada. Completed in August 2014, twenty people over a period of four weeks received either bexarotene or a placebo. Remarkably, the drug did appear to reduce amyloid, but only in the people who didn't have the APOE4 genotype. As Cummings scrutinised the data further, he reached two conclusions for that: 'It could be that it only works in APOE4 negative individuals,' he explained over the phone. 'Or, I think equally as likely, we may simply need to expose these people [to bexarotene] for longer, because the amyloid in APOE4 carriers is denser and more aggregated.'

Cummings is currently planning a second, year-long trial of bexarotene. Even if the drug fails to ameliorate the symptoms of dementia, it may plant the seeds for one that does. And a clever chemist, he argues, could theoretically remove the molecular components causing the potential side effects. Confident, innovative and reasonable, this approach to drug discovery reignited the hopes of clinicians and patients alike. So much so, in fact, that Cummings himself broke protocol and put three of his own patients on the drug. When I asked him if he'd seen any changes, he gently exhaled down the line. 'Well, one had very elevated triglycerides and so was only on it for a very short period of time. The other two continued for a few months and, you know, the families would do what they always do and say, "Oh, I think she's a little better," and then, "No, she's getting worse." In truth, I couldn't see a definitive pattern. You just can't know what's happening because it's such a slow disease and every patient has a slightly different course. So you cannot actually see whether you're helping them or not.'

Many of Cummings' patients have become personal friends. With their time slowly running out, with the stepwise manner of science ceaselessly rewriting the rules of Alzheimer's, they could not have asked for a more fearless pragmatist for their plight.

When I began investigating bexarotene I was hoping to have a more conclusive idea of whether it would work. But it is, as yet, unclear how this research story will end. In a broader sense, the fact that a cancer drug can twist the cogs of Alzheimer's inner gears says much about how we can approach the problem. It suggests that the web of causation stretches out into far more scientific domains than previously thought. Indeed, the stories of the last three chapters – of blood, prions and vision – vividly illustrate this point. While the challenge of describing Alzheimer's must be drawn on hard, clearly defined lines, the challenge of treating it must remain conceptually malleable. This is the conclusion researchers are now reaching, and as a result many have begun testing the impact of other seemingly unrelated drugs – such as statins (primarily aimed at reducing blood cholesterol), anti-epileptic drugs (principally aimed at minimising epileptic seizures) and incretin mimetics (predominantly aimed to treat type 2 diabetes). All show signs of ameliorating the effects of Alzheimer's in cell and animal models, and large-scale clinical trials are being discussed.

The web of treatment is widening.

PART V

Discovery

O N THE EVENING of 9 September 2012 Abbas went to sleep and never woke up. Aged eighty-two, his mind lost and his body frail, Abbas still needed help walking to the bathroom, and had a specially fitted hospital bed at his home in Tehran. His wife and three daughters, who'd been caring for him around the clock, stood ashen-faced as the doctor confirmed his death. After seven years of fear, confusion and profound loss, my grandfather was finally at peace.

My father flew to Iran the next day. He had known Abbas was not long for this world and admitted to being somewhat relieved: the father who no longer recognised his family had calmly slipped away in the night. It was the best he could hope for.

The doctors identified pneumonia as the cause of death. For all its cunning and unrelenting work, Alzheimer's isn't what kills in the end. People die from the complications of Alzheimer's: infected bedsores, broken skin and pneumonia can lead to sepsis and difficulty breathing; disorientation leads to a fatal fall; trouble swallowing makes a person choke on their food; some forget to eat altogether and suffer malnutrition. If a patient avoids all this, further complications set in, from stroke to heart disease to multiple organ failure. In its final act of forgetting, the brain forgets to tell the body how to stay alive.

For a long time my father didn't talk about Abbas's death. When I asked him why not, he said it was because he felt as if he hadn't done enough. He felt guilty as well as relieved. In many ways this is normal: guilt is a common product of grief, especially following the death of someone with Alzheimer's. After years of seeing a loved one's mind slowly disappear, it's often the carer's memories of exasperation and released frustration that come hurling back.

But my father's guilt came more from a feeling of inadequacy. He had been living and working in a foreign country for much of Abbas's decline, and therefore couldn't offer everything the family expected from a first-born son, which weighed heavily on him. He had seen television documentaries in which patients and relatives travel far and wide in search of answers. And now, looking back, he wished that he'd done the same. In researching this book, I thus made the decision to seek out researchers from the furthest corners of the earth and begin that search on his behalf.

I knew of several places that warranted exploration.

19

To the Ends of the Earth

What a piece of work is a man! How noble in reason, how infinite
in faculty! In form and moving how express and admirable!
In action how like an angel, in apprehension how like a god!
William Shakespeare, *Hamlet*

'EVERYBODY KNOWS DR Stefánsson,' said the driver as the taxi
lurched across the snow. A bitter Arctic wind caked the windows
in frost and a dimly lit sky hung overhead, the midday sun
barely above the horizon. I'd come to Reykjavík in Iceland: a small,
flat rock in the North Atlantic, whose inhabitants – not many, but
some – are virtually immune to Alzheimer's. How was this possible?
And what did it mean?

We pulled up at our destination. As I climbed out of the car,
the driver added: 'I haven't given him my DNA yet. But I will
soon!' To Icelanders, I would learn, this kind of talk was pretty
normal.

On an August day in 1996 a tall, Icelandic, exceedingly philosophical man named Kari Stefánsson had an idea. A neurologist and
pathologist, he'd seen countless Alzheimer's patients – both dead
and alive – and was beginning to tire of the slow, incremental and,
in his view, erroneous approach to the problem. Biologists, he
thought, could contemplate theories until the end of time, but they
still wouldn't have a concrete lead for drug companies to test. His

belief was that not enough attention had been paid to a simple yet unalterable truth: the brain is hard-wired by genetics. Differences in the sequence of DNA's four-letter code was the cardinal difference between Matthew and the wheat used at the Last Supper. It was the Holy Grail, Stefánsson insisted. And so, after twenty years toiling at American universities, he decided to return to Iceland with the singular purpose of eliminating common diseases by mining the genome of the Icelandic people.

It wasn't nearly as ridiculous as it sounds. With record low levels of immigration since the Vikings settled Iceland 1,100 years ago, the island's genetically homogenous population made it a unique natural laboratory. It was to Stefánsson what the Galapagos Islands were to Darwin. Unlike Darwin, however, Stefánsson was going to need a lot more than wits and a notebook. He wanted to collect and sequence the entire Icelandic genome, some 300,000 people. The cost would be enormous – certainly more than any money he could obtain publicly. And to make matters worse, it was illegal for an individual to create their own database on healthcare; many saw it as a disturbing, Orwellian prospect. So Stefánsson set up a private company, called DeCODE Genetics, and lobbied the Icelandic government to change the law.

He succeeded on both counts, and DeCODE immediately spread the word around Reykjavík and the wider community, asking anyone and everyone to give blood and/or saliva to help unlock the mysteries of human diseases. To ease the effort, the company sent out cheek swabs in the mail, telling people that a courier would come by to collect their sample, if they chose to give one. As an incentive, and to reach the remote villages outside the capital, the couriers were volunteers from the Icelandic Search and Rescue charity, which got a $20 donation for every sample it collected.

Not everyone was enamoured by Stefánsson's plan. Some saw it as an infringement of their private, most personal information. As one Icelandic journalist put it: 'It makes me very nervous . . . in Iceland everyone knows everyone and when you give your DNA sample, you are not just giving information about yourself.'[1] Stefánsson couldn't have disagreed more. The way he saw it, a healthcare system was only able to treat people by using the information amassed from previous generations. How was it fair, therefore, for anyone to take advantage of such a system and yet simultaneously refuse people the right to help improve that system for future generations?

He had a point. Critics had failed to appreciate that human samples were the lifeblood of medical advancements, not to mention optional and anonymous. Fortunately, many Icelanders did appreciate this. By 2004, 80,000 Icelanders had given samples; 120,000 by 2007, nearly half of Iceland's population. The DNA sequencers could hardly keep up. To cope with the deluge, DeCODE installed colossal freezers containing gigantic car-manufacturing robots (one freezer contained half a million vials of blood) and supercomputers capable of holding 20 petabytes of data. To put that into context, it's the equivalent of 10 billion floppy disks, or 10 trillion pages of text. But the usefulness of all that data paled in comparison to what turned out to be Iceland's most precious resource: genealogy.

Genealogy is a national obsession in Iceland. Almost every Icelandic saga begins with a lengthy description of family trees.[2] Here's one example: 'There was a man named Ulf, the son of Bjalfi and of Hallbera, the daughter of Ulf the Fearless. She was the sister of Hallbjorn Half-troll from Hrafnista, the father of Ketil Haeng . . .' And another: 'There was a man named Onund. He was the son of Ofeig Hobbler, whose father was Ivar Horse-cock. Onund's sister Gudbjorg was the mother of Gudbrand Lump, whose daughter Asta was the mother of King Olaf the Holy. On his mother's side . . .' And on it goes. Icelanders have done this for centuries. Stefánsson himself can trace his ancestry back to the Viking poet Egil Skallagrimsson, who lived in AD 900.

This record-keeping has proved essential for the DeCODE project. Since DNA is inherited in chunks of code – vast stretches of ATCG, rather than being passed down in individual 'letters'

– many Icelanders' genomes needn't be sequenced. They could simply be inferred by combining family trees with clever computers.

When Stefánsson put this strategy into action, the discoveries came in thick and fast. New genes underpinning heart attack, autism, schizophrenia and many cancers were unearthed, as well as genes influencing smoking behaviour, skin pigmentation and even creativity. The discoveries made headlines coast to coast, and Stefánsson was enshrined in *Time* magazine's top 100 people transforming the world. I remember the day I first heard about him. I was sitting in the lab, waiting for an experiment to finish, frustrated by how slow and inefficient academic research can often be. His success was bewitching. He was a maverick, a misfit, a rebellious pragmatist, unencumbered by politics and fully aware that curing big diseases requires big data and big capital. In 2012 the US pharmaceutical giant Amgen kept his dream alive by purchasing DeCODE for a little over $400 million. For Alzheimer's research, this was all a prologue to another vital clue.

On 2 August 2012 Stefánsson published data showing that about 1 per cent of 1,795 Icelanders carry a genetic mutation shielding them from Alzheimer's.[3] Astonishingly, it was found in APP, the same gene underlying Carol Jennings early-onset. But where Carol's mutation was due to a 'T' that should have been a 'C', the Icelanders' mutation was a 'T' that should have been an 'A'. This tiny genetic fluke had the effect of shifting beta-amyloid into reverse gear: while Carol's brain became saturated with amyloid, the Icelanders' brains produced *half* the usual amount. It was resounding support for John Hardy's amyloid hypothesis, and an olive branch to pharmaceutical developers, now weary of constantly having their fingers burned by this lead.

But the mutation also hinted at some deeper, primordial truths – about ageing and why Alzheimer's even existed.

'I'll give you an example of how strange memory is,' Stefánsson offered, seated in his spacious office at DeCODE's headquarters in the suburbs of Reykjavík, the imposing Hallgrímskirkja Church spire and craggy visage of Mount Esja visible from the window. 'When I was seven years old, I went to an old movie theatre located exactly where this building is. The movie was *The Scarlet Pimpernel*. Then, about thirty years later, I was in Chicago taking my daughter and her friend to the movies. On the way back, the following verse suddenly popped into my head: "Is he here or is he there, the French are seeking everywhere, is he in heaven or is he in hell, the elusive Scarlet Pimpernel". I haven't seen that movie since I was seven . . . Where does this come from?'

Just shy of seven feet, Stefánsson is a Herculean man, with ice-blue eyes and thick white hair. His father was an author and radio journalist, disappointed by his son's resolve to pursue science instead of writing. Stefánsson still remembers the summer night in 1968 when he and a classmate drank through the night, talking about life, purpose and the world of alternatives to choose from, before applying the very next day to medical school. Now, aged sixty-six, his childhood cinema recast as a genetics super-lab, he wakes every morning and comes into work feeling as if he's 'playing in the sandbox'.

He is an astute neurobiologist and a brilliant geneticist, but is one of the few people to stress how little we know about memory. 'We haven't the faintest idea how the brain generates memory. We don't even have a useful *definition* of memory. And you're going to write a book about a disease that assaults this function, but you cannot even define it! What the hell are you doing?' Again, he had a point. I'd become so wrapped up in trying to understand Alzheimer's that I'd swept the basic premise of what memory is under the rug.

'What about LTP and the synaptic network idea?' I countered. Wasn't this at least somewhere in the ballpark?

'What can I say?' he acknowledged with a shrug of ambivalence. 'It *sounds* reasonable. But my God is it magical.'

One of Stefánsson's trademark characteristics is his ability to view disease at the population level. Where many see a cruel and utterly meaningless defeat, Stefánsson sees the tragic but inevitable cost of evolution.

Take schizophrenia: in March 2015 DeCODE used the DNA of 86,000 Icelanders – plus a further 35,000 people from the Netherlands and Sweden – to show that schizophrenia and creativity actually share genetic roots.[4] The same genes underlying the disorder, it turns out, are also more common in painters, dancers, writers and musicians. So it isn't that you develop schizophrenia and therefore think differently, Stefánsson explained; it's much more likely that you think differently and therefore develop schizophrenia. Since the prevalence of schizophrenia is only 1 per cent worldwide, people with these genes have a roughly 10 per cent chance of developing the disorder. And this, he claims, is the small but striking price our species pays for the Mozarts, Shakespeares and Van Goghs of society.

A similar paradigm may exist for Alzheimer's owing to another special property of the Icelandic mutation: it protects against memory loss and cognitive decline in normal ageing, too. By using a cognitive test given to residents of Icelandic nursing homes, DeCODE found that people who carry the mutation are nearly eight times more likely to reach eighty-five as mentally sharp as they were at their peak. For Stefánsson, this is irrefutable proof that Alzheimer's is simply an accelerated form of ageing. 'What's often lost on people is that the brain is just an organ. And like everything else it's perishable. I mean, you look at yourself in the mirror in the morning and you see over the years that you change: your skin changes, your hair changes, your muscles change. Your brain changes as well. It deteriorates.

'I think Alzheimer's is somehow an expression of this fact. I mean, is it a design flaw when a disease terminates a life when we are relatively old, or is it a masterpiece in the design? That depends on how you look at it. It depends on whether you look at it from the point of view of the individual, or the point of view of the species.'

'Assuming that's true, what evolutionary bill is Alzheimer's footing?' I asked. 'Or is that the wrong question?'

'This is exactly the right question,' Stefánsson replied. 'We're born to have offspring and die. What our roles are beyond that is beyond me. I don't know why we last this long. But there is some data to indicate that the Grandmother Effect is real.'

The Grandmother Effect is a fascinating theory. Formulated by anthropologists in the late 1990s, it argues that the reason grandmothers live many years after menopause is to help daughters with childcare. It was the Hadza hunter-gatherer tribe in Tanzania who first lent credence to the idea; researchers found that mothers in the tribe have more children if their own mothers helped raise them. (Grandfathers, by contrast, can stay fertile until they die and so the explanation for their longevity is that it's either for them to continue mating, or that it's some kind of genetic side effect of female longevity.)

It goes without saying that child-rearing demands grandmothers be mentally sound, certainly Alzheimer's-free, and today evolutionary biologists are uncovering genes responsible for exactly that. One such gene, CD33, was found in our closest relative, the chimpanzee. Intriguingly, though, this gene only grants mind-protective status when it's found in humans. And since chimps and other primates usually die once their fertility ends, it's possible that genes like this have evolved solely in humans to make the Grandmother Effect a reality. As the distinguished Indian physician Ajit Varki told a journalist in 2015: 'Grandmothers are so important, we've even evolved genes to protect their minds.'[5]

Still, Stefánsson is no fatalist about ageing and Alzheimer's. Even if ageing is 'paid for' by Alzheimer's, we have still evolved minds to eradicate the illness. Before getting to the knotty issue of treatment, however, I wanted to know what he thought about the influence of stress, diet, education and sleep – the topics still fresh in my mind.

He took a dim view. 'I think there's no solid evidence for any of these. There *have* to be environmental factors for Alzheimer's, and whether it proceeds slowly or fast, but I honestly don't know what they are.'

It wasn't the answer I wanted to hear. Then again, much of what I'd learned was an answer I didn't want to hear; it was almost becoming a sign of the truth. In any case, lifestyle measures were a low-hanging fruit. Iceland's real gift was the message it sent to the pharmaceutical industry.

Around the time Big Pharma was testing amyloid immunisation in clinical trials, vast swathes of neuroscientists were devising a back-up plan. What if, they thought, instead of trying to rid the brain of amyloid, we prevented it from ever arising in the first place – like in the brains of Icelanders with the mutation?

Since the discovery that amyloid was merely the by-product of a normal protein – the amyloid precursor protein, APP – questions were asked about what the APP protein was actually doing in the brain. Beyond sitting at a neuron's surface, with one end jutting inside the cell and the other out, no one really knew. Perhaps it was just another run-of-the-mill signalling molecule, a 'sedan' on the grand intercellular highway of brain chemistry. Whatever its purpose, it certainly had a routine: first an enzyme chopped off a large piece of it, which then allowed a second, smaller piece to be released from the neuron. Although I should say *unleashed*, for this small piece was beta-amyloid, the substance of plaques.

In 1999 five independent groups of scientists identified this chopping enzyme. They called it BACE (beta-site APP-cleaving enzyme).[6] It turned out that Carol Jennings's genetic mutation caused BACE to ramp up its activity, which had the effect of churning out beta-amyloid much faster than normal. It was akin to a faulty traffic light stuck on green – and too many sedans were getting through. So scientists looked into the possibility of blocking BACE and redressing the balance.

The results were not encouraging. From 2003 to 2011 a tide of animal tests unveiled serious side effects. Mice genetically engineered to lack the enzyme suffered blindness, seizures, spine abnormalities and memory problems to boot. Switching BACE off was clearly not ideal. What about chemically restraining it? In 2011 E-Lilly was among the first to try this tack. The 'BACE-inhibitor compounds', as they became known, were certainly better, but blindness remained a vexing fly in the ointment.

Still, progress of a kind.

So Lilly kept at it, tweaking and retweaking the recipe until the animals finally appeared normal. Compound LY2886721 was the coveted batch. It produced no side effects and yet, crucially, reduced beta-amyloid formation in the animals' brains. A success! The company immediately moved to human trials. Upon giving forty-seven healthy volunteers daily doses of the drug for a fortnight, everything looked fine. Emboldened, Lilly funded a six-month Phase two trial in 130 cases of mild Alzheimer's.

Here, you guessed it, is where things went wrong. An undisclosed number of patients showed signs of liver damage. Not wanting to take any chances, Lilly immediately terminated the trial. Merck, another US pharmaceutical company, picked up the baton. Their drug, dubbed MK-8931, made it through eighty-eight healthy volunteers with no side effects. And so they cautiously pressed on. Despite Merck's headway, however, the message in the pharmaceutical industry was clear: invest elsewhere.

One could hardly blame them. Between 2000 and 2012, of the 244 Alzheimer's drugs tested in 413 clinical trials, only one was approved (Namenda™, a drug similar to the acetylcholinesterase inhibitors, and similarly insufficient). In total, the drug candidates racked up a lamentable 99.6 per cent failure rate – even higher than cancer, at 81 per cent.[7] Our unsophisticated grasp of the disease, combined with the dizzying cost of drug development – it costs about $100 million per trial; over $2 billion all-in – made Alzheimer's drugs, in the words of one pharmaceutical chemist, 'almost perfectly set up for expensive failures'.[8] The reluctance for renewed attempts almost seemed a fait accompli.

But then something magical happened. Further detective work

at DeCODE revealed that the Icelanders' protective gene caused their BACE enzyme to reduce its activity. In other words, the mutation was a natural BACE inhibitor. If that wasn't proof this lead was worth pursuing, nothing was.

Wide-eyed and reinvigorated, Big Pharma returned to the table. And to share the risk, they teamed up: Lilly joined forces with AstraZeneca, the British–Swedish pharmaceutical giant, pledging a whopping $500 million to co-develop a new BACE inhibitor; Eisai, the Japanese company, struck a deal with the US company Biogen; and Swiss-led Novartis partnered with Amgen. The abundance of heavyweight competition marked a momentous victory for Alzheimer's research.

Hungry for a release date, I rang every company.

'We're talking somewhere between five and ten years,' said Sasha Kamb, Amgen's Vice-President of Discovery Research. 'DeCODE has proved that this idea should work, so I think the only question left is: when do we need to intervene and by how much?'

Ricardo Dolmetsch, Global Head of Neuroscience at Novartis, was even more optimistic. 'Between three and eight years. I think Kari Stefánsson's data provided the nail in the coffin that beta-amyloid is important and that if you inhibit BACE that would be a good thing.'

The most cautious estimate I got during these prying exchanges was from a representative for Eisai. 'Seven to twelve years,' she had said, not exactly bursting the bubble.

As to whether they will work, I kept something Stefánsson had told me fresh in my mind. 'They're going to be spectacular,' he'd said.

Driving through the barren lava fields of the Reykjavík peninsula, en route to the airport, I mulled over Stefánsson's special role in the abolition of Alzheimer's. No doubt he was another William Summers, another outlier, only one with the formidable power of genetics on his side. When his contribution would actually help people like my grandfather, Arnold, Carol, Marie, Victoria, Li and Pam, I couldn't say. Big Pharma's projections seemed ambitious, but I vowed to remain optimistic.

Looking out of the window, at the flat expanse of all-consuming darkness, I suddenly glimpsed the fleeting glow of a streetlight puncturing the polar night. For a brief moment I could see the snow was melting.

Spring was coming.

20

Insights from India

Where the mind is without fear and the head is held high,
Where knowledge is free,
Where the world has not been broken up into fragments
By narrow domestic walls,
Where words come out from the depth of truth,
Where tireless striving stretches its arms towards perfection,
Where the clear stream of reason has not lost its way
Into the dreary desert sand of dead habit,
Where the mind is led forward by thee
Into ever-widening thought and action,
Into that heaven of freedom, my Father, let my country awake.
                    Rabindranath Tagore, *Gitanjali*, 1912

THE WHITE-ROBED MAN hands me a cup of chai while the midday sun pelts his calloused fingers. This is Hari Chand, a farmer in the village of Shahpur Kalan, in Ballabgarh, northern India. His ninety-four years of age asserts his status as village elder. And he's not alone: nearby, several more elders stoop on wooden benches to smoke the customary hookah pipe, quietly chatting while offering me looks of curious bemusement.

Ballabgarh is a patchwork of twenty-eight villages located some thirty-five kilometres south of New Delhi. Its elderly inhabitants are mostly illiterate, impoverished farmers, many of whom have never left the village. I'm here to retrace the steps of a sixteen-year investigation, which started in 1988, when the US National Institute on Aging set out to widen the net for Alzheimer's clues:

> Other countries, cultures, ethnic or population groups, with different exposures and habits, may offer clues to the [cause] of the disease that are not apparent in Western industrialized nations. The need to search more aggressively and widely for potent modifiable risk factors requires movement beyond national boundaries.[1]

Looking around, I'm hard-pressed to think of a more suitable candidate for such an objective. Many of the villagers are bone thin; clearly malnourished. They live in crumbling sugar-cube houses or wooden shacks covered with corrugated metal sheets. They burn cow dung for fuel. Electricity is a luxury few possess. And water is supplied by a single cement basin and a few rusty pumps. But another difference seemed to be their resistance to dementia. Sporadic reports from New Delhi's Centre for Ageing Research suggested that Alzheimer's was 'unusual' in this part of India, that plaque and tangle pathology were 'rarely found' post-mortem.

'My memory is good,' Chand said proudly. 'I think there are some people in Ballabgarh who don't want to remember certain things, but I've never heard of anyone having problems with their memory.' Chand has farmed these fields since he was ten years old. His memory stretches as far back as his teenage years, to the arguments his mother and father had when they had to borrow money to pay the British colonialists' high taxes. Having retired at the age of eighty-five, Chand now spends his days in the company of his ten children, eight grandchildren and seven great-grandchildren. After reeling off all their names for me, he said that I'm not the first scientist to visit his town. Others had come with similar questions, not so long ago.

Leading the NIA study was Mary Ganguli, an Indian-born psychiatrist at the University of Pittsburgh, Pennsylvania (in collaboration with Vijay Chandra and colleagues at the Centre for Ageing

Research and the Department of Community Medicine of the All India Institute of Medical Sciences). She had her work cut out. The study required a group of elderly people in a region where many don't know their real age, family histories in a community where medical records are virtually non-existent, and cognitive tests in an area where few have ever put pen to paper or kept track of the Roman or Hindu calendar. It moved us from the realm of telephones and bank accounts to the era of spirits and storytelling around the fire. It was, at heart, a radical act of learning by unlearning, advancing by retreating.

'They have the same cognitive functions as educated people,' Ganguli explained over the phone. 'It's just about finding a reasonable way to tap them. It's important because we might have learned all we're going to learn, or most of what we're going to learn, by only studying the risk factors for dementia among white people in wealthy countries.'

To overcome the cultural and educational disparity, Ganguli's team devised 'culture-fair' tests of cognition. Since the villagers speak a phonetic dialect of Hindi, for example, they were asked to repeat certain sounds instead of reading or writing things down. Questions involving abstract mental arithmetic, like the subtracting seven task I did in chapter four, were personalised to questions about rupees and village bus fares. As an adaptation of the standard task 'Write a sentence', the researchers instead asked participants 'Tell me something' – anything to gauge their ability to generate a complete thought.

A bewildered 'What shall I tell you?' was a common response, often leading, Ganguli wrote, to 'awkward and pointless exchanges between interviewer and subject'. The experience resulted in the final version being 'Tell me something about your house.' Even the idea of taking a test was alien to many of them. When asked to memorise a list of words, most villagers simply laughed and asked, 'What for?' When told a story and asked to repeat it, many would say, 'You call that a story? Let me tell you a story!' before proceeding to embellish the original tale with great dramatic flair. When the interviewers insisted they follow the rules, they often replied, with sincere wonder, 'Why?'

At one point the team tried something called the Boston Naming Test, a neuropsychological exam where the candidate is shown line drawings of various objects – a boat, a whistle, a kangaroo – and asked to name them. But the objects were completely unfamiliar to the villagers. Some even had difficulty with the concept of a drawing, and started grasping at the paper itself for more insight. So Ganguli decided to use 3-D models instead. One was a miniature model tree, which a member of her team had purchased in a children's museum back in Pittsburgh. To avoid confusion, he'd cut the wooden base off before posting it to Ganguli.

'Okay, what's this?' she asked when she presented it to them.

'Broccoli,' came the reply.

A different approach was clearly needed, and so she decided to focus on her subjects' ability to perform normal day-to-day business. Not too much is expected of these elderly citizens – cooking, working the fields and tending the fire are all done by younger family members. Daughters-in-law are especially required to look after them. 'At a certain age, many of the women hand over the pantry keys to their eldest daughter,' Ganguli explained, 'and then sit back and relax. They become ladies of leisure, if they can afford it, if there are enough daughters to do all the work.'

But these weather-beaten seniors do have some responsibilities, like watching over grandchildren, and overseeing festivals and marriages; so the team devised a new scoring system based on questions such as, 'Does he express his opinion on important family matters?', 'Is she able to remember important festivals such as Holi, Diwali?', 'Does he ever lose his way in the village?' The results confirmed what many had already declared. There was a curiously low level of Alzheimer's in the village.

It was the BBC that first alerted me to this story. In February 2010 it ran an article headlined INDIAN VILLAGE MAY HOLD KEY TO BEATING DEMENTIA, in which the remarkably wholesome lifestyle of Ballabgarh's residents was pointed to as the reason for their low rates. 'The people of Ballabgarh are unusually healthy,' it announced. 'It is a farming community, so most of them are very physically active and most eat a low-fat vegetarian diet. Obesity is virtually unheard of. Life in this fertile farming community is also low in stress, and family support is still strong, unlike in other, more urban parts of India.'

But Ganguli told a different story. Despite all the effort that had gone into carefully developing the assessment tools, her instinct was that something was off – that an elusive, protective agent, somehow camouflaged amid the vicissitudes of Ballabgarhian life, was wishful thinking. There were too many 'what ifs'; too few absolutes. The villagers' diet, for instance, consists mainly of whole-wheat flatbreads, lentils, vegetables and yoghurt. Since everyone in the village eats this, whether it makes any difference is impossible to say. The idea of a stress-free life in Ballabgarh also seems fanciful. The villagers' livelihood hinges on a capricious climate, with drought and crop failures giving Indian farming a notoriously high suicide rate. Indeed, during my visit, Chand explained how the Indian government is further assaulting their livelihood by buying the farmland cheap and urbanising it for foreign investors. Only by increasing their yield can they hope to survive as an industry – and so every day, said Chand, they pray, nerve-racked, that 'the gods give the rain'.

To this day Ganguli has mulled over what else it could be. Whether or not physical activity protects them is another unknown, not assessed by the study – though Ganguli lends more credence to this possibility than any other. 'It's quite possible. They're an active community. They walk everywhere. They don't have cars. When they were younger many of them worked the fields, which is hard physical labour, so that might be protective.' Chand told me he spent ten to twelve hours a day ploughing the fields; sometimes his family even slept in the fields. 'And we know that everything that's good for the heart is good for the brain. The trouble is – and I'm sure you've come across this – Alzheimer's pathology begins in our brain when we are much younger, decades before symptoms start. So we would need to perform a trial where we make half the younger villagers follow the same exercise protocol for the next forty or fifty years to see if it really reduces their risk.'

Genetics might play a role. Ganguli's team genotyped more than 4,000 villagers – aged fifty-five to ninety-five – and found that the APOE4 gene is rare here compared to more developed parts of the world. But even this explanation had pitfalls: APOE4 increases the risk of heart disease as well; did the APOE4 carriers die of heart disease before they could get symptoms of Alzheimer's? Which begged another question. Was this all just a function of India's low life expectancy, which according to the latest average is sixty-two?

To understand the answer, it's important to know the difference between disease prevalence and disease incidence. Prevalence is the proportion of people at any given time with the condition: a kind of snapshot of a population. Incidence is the rate at which new cases of disease occur in the population over a defined period of time: one year, for instance. The relationship between incidence and prevalence is duration, and for Alzheimer's, it's duration of survival. Two populations might therefore have the same incidence of Alzheimer's but prevalence would be higher in the population that lives longer.

In the west, we maintain elderly people in good health, meaning they can live a long time with dementia. In India and other developing nations, however, cultural influences can preclude this kind of sustained healthcare. The children often keep their parents at home, do all the housework, feed them, wash them and nurse them if they get sick. As Chand's eldest son explained to me, 'From when we first start walking, from the very first time our parents hold our hand, it is our duty to look after them. When they get old, they need *our* hand, our support – no matter how sick they become. This is our culture.' Rather than being a product of low life expectancy, then, it's possible that underreporting, due to the low expectations of Ballabgarh's elders and the unparalleled level of respect and care they receive from the young, may have concealed many cases of Alzheimer's from Ganguli's study.

I liked the way Ganguli viewed this riddle. It reminded me of something I'd almost forgotten. Science is messy, its tools forever incomplete. In the lab we're largely cocooned from this. Everything comes neatly packaged in IKEA-style kits. If something doesn't work, it's usually the fault of the scientist. And when a tool isn't up to the challenge, we often just wait for one that is. We push boundaries from the comfort of clearly defined lines. But Ganguli and her team scrapped all that. They were going back to basics, back to the styles of Joseph Priestley and Alfred Russel Wallace – intrepid explorers, poking in the dark for the eurekas only this approach can dispense.

She mentioned a similar study, carried out in 1995, in which researchers compared Alzheimer's prevalence between African Americans living in Indianapolis and Nigerian Africans in the city of Ibadan, Nigeria.[2] The contrast was powerful for essentially neutralising genetic differences – the African Americans had migrated to America during the slave trade 200 years earlier, which is arguably not enough time for intermarriages to outweigh environmental influences. Lo and behold, Alzheimer's prevalence was lower in Nigeria than in Indianapolis. Again, nobody really knows why. Evidently something in the environment is at play.

Another report, published a few years earlier by the same group, supports that suspicion. They looked at a population of Cree Indians in Winnipeg, Manitoba.[3] It may be Canada, but the native Cree live in sovereign reservations with a culture and tradition all of their own. Most of the men continue to hunt and fish well into old age. Many of the women maintain an interest in elaborate crafts like sculpting and quillwork. They still embrace modern society (the buffalo-hide tipis are just for show) and yet the prevalence of Alzheimer's remains unusually low. If an undiscovered guardian is somewhere in their environment, the most 'striking impression', the report noted, was the 'continuity of activities of the elderly Native subjects'. Keep active, in other words. Stay busy.

The rejection of cultural differences has consequences, too. A

1996 study published by the National Institute on Aging, entitled 'Prevalence of dementia in older Japanese-American men in Hawaii', found that elderly Japanese people living in America have higher rates of Alzheimer's than those living in Japan.[4] Nearly 4,000 participants aged seventy-one to ninety-three were involved, impressive even by today's standards. Though the cause of the discrepancy was never determined, researchers largely attribute it to the western diet – especially because Alzheimer's rates in Japan have shot up since the gradual westernisation of the country's diet. 'Genetics loads the gun, lifestyle pulls the trigger' is a popular biology adage. It reconciles the argument over nature versus nurture, and each of these studies is a stark reminder of it.

Before I left Ballabgarh, I saw another group of elders sitting in a circle beneath a wooden shelter. They were playing card games, laughing merrily while their children worked in the acres of paddy fields around them. In spite of so much uncertainty, it definitely seemed that they were doing something right.

While the search for that 'something' continues, research into the ancient Indian spice turmeric, commonly used in curry powder, has flourished. This spice, derived from the roots of *Curcuma longa*, a yellow flowering plant native to the monsoon forests of South East Asia, possesses surprising therapeutic properties that may help explain India's low Alzheimer's rates.

In the early 2000s nutritionists noticed that turmeric's most active ingredient, a compound known as curcumin, dismantles beta-amyloid plaques in a petri dish.[5] A few years later, Fusheng Yang, a neurologist at the University of California Los Angeles, fed curcumin to Alzheimer's mice and showed that it does indeed enter the brain and destroy plaques.[6] Further tests found that curcumin might even stop tangles forming. Following this work, in 2013, Muaz Belviranli at Selçuk University, Turkey, demonstrated that curcumin fed to old rats improved their spatial memory and reduced the cellular damage associated with ageing.[7] To date, there are more than 1,000 published studies with similar findings, and researchers have spent the last decade eagerly trying to reproduce the effects in humans.

The results, unfortunately, remain speculative. In 2006 researchers at the National University of Singapore tested 1,010 elderly Asians – Chinese, Malays and Indians – aged sixty to ninety-three, and discovered that those who ate curry 'often or very often' scored higher on cognitive tests than those who 'never or rarely' did.[8] But with such a vast age range and diverse ethnic mix it's hard to rule out other influences. The data from Alzheimer's patients has been equally ambiguous, with only a few studies showing positive effects. Nevertheless, since most human studies have measured curcumin's effect in months, not years, the evidence from cell and animal models needn't be dismissed. In fact many scientists believe the prime obstacle is the spice's transience: since curcumin doesn't absorb well into blood (over 60 per cent is excreted in stool) the question remains whether it would have an impact if its blood levels could be raised and maintained.

Mark Taylor, a chemist at the University of Lancaster, England, is now trying to develop methods to bind curcumin on to the surface of nanoparticles: a form of nanotechnology made using molecules of fats, proteins, iron, even gold.[9] This so-called *nano-curcumin* will hopefully increase curcumin's absorption in the body, allowing more of it to reach the brain and work its magic. If it ever is concluded that curcumin guards Ballabgarh's population from Alzheimer's, we shall look back in wonderment at the measures we employed to mimic something so simple.

As it happens, Chand and his elderly companions consume turmeric often. In India the average consumption of curcumin is 80–200 milligrams per day (I myself can't remember the last time I ate a meal containing the ingredient). In clinical trials researchers used doses of up to 4 grams a day for six to twelve months. When compared to a lifetime of cultural habit, though, even this dose might be too little too late, and so it's difficult to draw any firm conclusions about curcumin's therapeutic value – larger, lengthier, more sophisticated trials are required. But still, Ganguli told me the evidence is encouraging, and she's as sceptical by nature as they come.

This story speaks to a higher truth not mentioned enough. Science doesn't seek to prove hypotheses; it seeks to disprove them. Every finding has scores of older, closely related findings trailing behind, each having been disproved, amending the scientific narrative. Even completely new discoveries must be fallible in some way, ready to be updated when a better idea comes along. Science orbits the truth; it doesn't live there. The twentieth-century philosopher Karl Popper understood this better than anyone. He's famous for proclaiming that a discovery 'must be falsifiable: and in so far as it is not falsifiable, it does not speak about reality'.[10] But I've always preferred something else he said: 'Science must begin with myths, and with the criticism of myths.' Is the feeling that Chand's and the other elders' lifestyle protects them from Alzheimer's just that − a feeling, speculation, a myth?

Possibly. Only when Ganguli and others have falsified and criticised enough will we know for certain. But that scientists are now combing the world for answers fills me with hope. It shows just how far we are willing to go.

21

Clues from Colombia

Nature never draws a line without smudging it.

Sir Winston Churchill,
Great Contemporaries, 1937

T HE PLANE TOUCHED down with a gentle thud and slowed
to greet the terminals of José María Córdova Airport. I
collected my suitcase and caught a bus heading north-west
to Medellín, the second-largest city in Colombia. This is a country
of coffee-lovers and football fanatics and fierce national pride. It's
also home to the largest population of Alzheimer's victims on the
planet.

Over three centuries, some 5,000 people spread among twenty-
five Colombian families have been affected. They have what the
locals call *La Bobera* – the foolishness. In reality, they possess a
genetic mutation that's now recognised as the most common cause
of early-onset Alzheimer's: the Paisa mutation, named after the
people of the region. This cursed mishap of DNA sprang from
obscurity to global recognition in 1996, after being identified by a
team of US researchers.[1] But it was a young Colombian neurologist named Francisco Lopera who found the families, and risked
much to help them.

As a trainee neurologist at Medellín's University of Antioquia,
Lopera wasn't quite sure where his interests lay. Then, one day in
1984, a forty-seven-year-old man from Belmira, a sleepy town in
the nearby mountains, walked into Lopera's office with a bizarre

tale. He had been struck by an unnatural memory loss, he told Lopera. The man – let's call him Mr Rodríguez – believed it was the *maldición*, an evil spell that now befell nine others in his family. He'd been to see the local witch doctors for various potions and tonics, but they hadn't worked. He sought Lopera's help as a last resort, for many in the town remained superstitious and believed it was a form of paranormal retribution. The family must have done something wicked, they thought. Perhaps they had touched the 'bad tree', or stolen from the church. But Lopera urged Rodríguez to dismiss such claims, and travelled with him to Belmira to examine the rest of the family.

When he returned, Lopera still wasn't sure about the diagnosis. Shortly after, however, he was visited by a woman of the same age from another mountain town, called Angostura, where seventy people were affected with the same thing. Then fourteen more surfaced in the town of Yarumal, less than twenty kilometres away.

Lopera didn't as yet know it was Alzheimer's. That certitude arrived in 1995, when a man from Angostura donated his brain to the university and Lopera, together with Alison Goate (our heroine geneticist from chapter five) found that not only was it filled with plaques and tangles, but it also harboured another genetic mutation to add to the growing list.

With that, Lopera informed every family of the *maldición*'s true cause. He told them to expect many scientists from America and beyond to visit their secluded homes. By giving blood samples and having memory tests, he said, they would be helping themselves and the research into a disease that was, to their astonishment, currently enveloping the globe.

But this wasn't Carol Jennings's living room. Guerrilla warfare was a material problem in this part of Colombia. The FARC, a left-wing terrorist group, had been drug trafficking and murdering people for the past fifty years. Their 'revolutionary' methods involved kidnapping, attacking civilians, using child soldiers, and assassinating indigenous people – all of which strangled Colombia's growth into a prosperous and free society. In some areas the violence was so bad that many people fled into the outskirts of Medellín itself. Lopera took every precaution he could, often sending scouts ahead to gather families on the quiet.

It didn't always work, of course. During one excursion a nurse was kidnapped by guerrillas and detained for eight days. Incredibly, she was released and permitted to continue when the guerrilla chief realised that his own mother had Alzheimer's. But such mitigation only extended so far, and so Lopera and his team stopped visiting towns like Angostura for years. Only in the mid-2000s did the scientists venture out once more, when conservative President Álvaro Uribe – whose own father was murdered by the FARC – used the military to force the guerrillas into retreat (today, Uribe's policies have made it safe for foreign investment in Colombia, tremendously improving the country's economy). Finally, Lopera could ascertain enough data to turn *La Bobera* into one of the world's most enlightening groups of Alzheimer's patients.

Carlos Díaz was among them. When he wasn't fixing cars as the local mechanic, he was polishing his favourite truck and watching football with his two sons and four daughters. His wife Maria knew him as a man of strong work ethic and high spirits; but when Carlos turned forty-seven, everything changed. 'He started looking at me like he was lost,' Maria told me at her home in the hills bordering Medellín. I had travelled there with Lucía Madrigal, a psychologist who's worked with Lopera since the beginning, and Gabriel Aristizábal, my translator. 'One day, he went outside to clean his truck, and walked twenty-five blocks away. If we hadn't searched for him he'd probably be in the middle of the mountains. To be honest, I thought it was something supernatural. Weird things were happening in the house: the lights were going off, things kept moving from place to place. So I just took care of him, because he wasn't a difficult patient.'

Maria emitted a distinct calm – a toughness, an armour – that quickly explained itself. In the next room, Maria's forty-five-year-old daughter, Alejandra, was being informed of my visit. She too has Alzheimer's – as did one of her sisters, Camila, who died a month earlier. Providence has yet to reveal who else in the family has Alzheimer's. Six of Carlos's twelve siblings had been affected, and all had become sick in their mid-forties. But while Maria now accepts it as a disease, her sons cannot. When Camila died, they persuaded their sisters to change religion – from Catholic to Protestant – in the hope that whatever spirit was tormenting the family would now be appeased, allowing the illness to die with Camila.

As Maria spoke, Alejandra appeared in the doorway and slowly walked in to sit opposite me. She'd been outside talking to Madrigal, who later told me that Alejandra had recently become volatile, even aggressive. A few days earlier, she'd tried to strangle her mother, and so it was important to assess her mood before introducing me. Not that Alejandra looked particularly dangerous. Baby-faced and doe-eyed, she looked at me with curiosity rather than suspicion.

'I try my best here,' she said to me in a stifled whisper, before asking, 'Why is this happening inside my brain? The doctor says it's because I'm changing . . . Yesterday I was thinking some things, and then suddenly, everything blanked . . . Is this correct? Is this normal?' I assured her that scientists were doing everything they could. She returned a look I could not quite decipher: a frozen stare suggesting neither apprehension nor confusion. Gabriel repeated what I had said using different words, but it was as if he too needed a translator to bridge the divide. Although her memory was failing, language was clearly Alejandra's most pressing concern.

After a long silence she said, 'Okay . . . I'm so sorry. The words are about to come . . . but they do not come . . . it's like I have a gum, and the words get stuck to it . . . I want to speak well again . . . I want my words to get out like vomit; vomiting is easy, but the words are not.' Then she looked directly at me. 'I think about myself as a baby, like a baby trying to learn again. That's how I feel.'

E280A, the Paisa mutation, is thought to have entered Colombia through Spanish immigration; thirteen of the twenty-five families can be traced back to a Spanish conquistador in the seventeenth century.[2] The mutation carriers are unique for a number of reasons. Some patients experience epilepsy, as well as a movement disorder called cerebral ataxia. They have an especially hard time remembering faces. And they become filled with what are known as 'cotton wool' plaques – large, ball-like structures that completely dislodge neighbouring brain regions. Moreover, imaging of their brains reveals an eye-catching *hyper*activation of the hippocampus, visible years before memories fade, as if the hippocampus knows what's coming and kicks into overdrive to protect itself, although if and how Paisa mutation-carriers perceive this is unknown. Education doesn't appear to delay the symptoms; it merely leads to an earlier diagnosis. And they decline rapidly, often dying within four years instead of the average eight to ten.

Carlos was only fifty when he died. In the months preceding his death he was mostly bedbound but could sometimes be found sitting in a corner, chewing raw sugar cane. When I asked Madrigal if these families were getting any extra help from the government, she laughed.

'No,' she said. 'Welcome to Latin America.'

'Look at this.' Lopera spun in his chair and turned the computer screen towards me. 'We've found that Paisa mutation-carriers show brain changes and signs of the Alzheimer's in their blood as young as nine years old. As *children*.' He spoke in a slow, lilting Spanish accent, and exuded a warm-heartedness I've come to expect from Colombians. (When I'd contacted him for the interview, he sent me a week-long agenda of patient visits and lab tours.) There was something intimate about the way he spoke of the Colombian families, too. Maybe it was his youth spent in similar circumstances: the son of a farmer and one of sixteen siblings facing stark poverty and an uncertain future. 'With this kind of population,' he continued, 'we can study the natural evolution of the disease before the brain is completely destroyed.'

Lopera now finds himself in a unique position. For the purpose of testing new drugs, the Colombian cohort has become the envy of scientists around the world. Nowhere else are so many people, all densely packed within the same locale, unambiguously bound for Alzheimer's. It was more than a natural laboratory; it was a natural manufacturing complex. Among the first to recognise this were the California-based biotech firm Genentech and the Banner Alzheimer's Institute in Arizona. In 2013 they began a five-year prevention study using a drug called Crenezumab – a new anti-body designed to clear multiple forms of amyloid. If it works, the Colombians will be the first to receive it. 'We'd be giving people at the highest imminent risk of Alzheimer's access to treatment they wouldn't otherwise have,' Eric Reiman, executive director of the Banner Alzheimer's Institute, told the *New York Times*.[3]

Many participants are in their thirties, an age bracket Lopera considers viable for prevention trials. Like Henrik Zetterberg and now many others, he thinks that most clinical trials have been an exercise in shutting the stable door after the horse has bolted. 'The biggest problem with Alzheimer's research is that the pharmaceutical industry is primarily testing drugs in the clinical phase, when you don't have much of a brain left. We need to work here' – he pointed to an image of a thirty-year-old brain that showed sparse deposits of amyloid – 'when the brain is more or less healthy.'

Like many researchers, Lopera's strategy is early detection using Henrik Zetterberg's time-travelling biomarkers from chapter eight, followed by an intense regimen of amyloid therapy. The beauty of his trial is that a negative outcome would be almost as valuable as a positive one. This is because he knows, unequivocally, that if Crenezumab fails, it's got something to do Crenezumab, not the trial candidates. Having so much wiggle room means he can also be more creative, and his next objective is to examine Paisa children, ranging from eight to sixteen years old, in order to build a timeline of Alzheimer's unlike any other.

When I left Lopera I made a note to touch base with him in a few years. The never-ending uncertainty of my quest often left me feeling as if I were chasing a shadow. But his is a quest with a concrete ending.

The next day I left Medellín and made for the mountains. Winding up a steep and tortuous road – Gabriel driving while he and Madrigal talked Colombian politics – we were heading to Belmira, home to the first known Paisa-mutation family. This is dairy farming terrain, where cows and white Spanish bungalows dot the landscape and the sunlight, hitting the earth directly, makes the hills and everything around a brighter, almost luminescent green. We drove past motor-cyclists hauling precarious loads and *chivas* (colourful buses without windows) ferrying people between towns. Wooden crosses and statues of the Virgin Mary were everywhere, and at 2,600 metres above sea level, a limitless vista of the city took shape below.

Within two hours we had arrived in Belmira, a cluster of rough-hewn houses standing around a tall church, deep beneath the sharp, flora-laden slopes of the Andes. Walking through a small wooden gate, we were greeted by six dogs and eight cats and a short, bull-necked man pushing his way through them. Forty-seven-year-old Miguel Rodríguez lives here with his wife and two children. Home for the Rodríguez family is a wide, single-storey collection of rooms, each adorned with rosaries and Catholic memorabilia, separated by a large open courtyard. The garden was festooned with potted flowers, and strips of land where the family grow potatoes, corn, carrots and coriander.

Miguel started developing severe symptoms three years ago. He and his twelve siblings are the offspring of Mr Rodríguez, Lopera's first patient. So far, one sibling has died of the disease, and two others are currently sick. I shook Miguel's hand and apologised, in Spanish, for my poor Spanish. He smiled broadly and released a mirthful laugh. His wife, Laura, then appeared and showed us into the sitting room. She had to guide Miguel to his chair; he moved with a shuffling gait and seemed quite unaware of his surroundings. Laura, now forty-five, was nineteen when she married Miguel. She said that he worked with livestock and never complained about his health. She first noticed the illness when he began talking to himself in the mirror and repeating himself in conversation. One day, she recalled, he had a cold and was wiping his nose, but the second he put the tissue in his pocket, he immediately brought it back out to use again; the cycle was so incessant she had to take it off him to prevent a nose rash.

'When he wakes up in the morning, he forgets where the bathroom is,' she said, while of the rest of the family huddled inside. Two of Miguel's brothers were here, as were his son, daughter and new daughter-in-law. He appeared vaguely aware that our conversation was about him, but Laura assured me this wasn't a problem. Looking at me with a sort of quizzical affection, he suddenly pointed to a framed picture of Jesus Christ hanging on the wall.

'He's the boss.'

'I know,' I said, smiling.

Laura continued. 'He's becoming a little aggressive.'

'That's a lie,' Miguel instantly responded.

'Sometimes I don't understand what he's saying—'

'No, no, no,' he proclaimed.

'What do you like to do now?' I asked, wanting to keep the mood light.

'I work . . . I go to my job . . . That's it,' he replied, still smiling.

Laura shook her head. 'He stopped working five years ago. Now he just sits around and sleeps. He's quite easy. Sometimes he gets lost.'

'I cannot stand it,' their daughter, Isabel, added. 'My dad was really happy. He laughed with everyone. He loved playing football. But now he can't do anything.'

Miguel's younger brother, Daniel, weighed in. 'It's cruel and sad, because there's nothing for the family, and they're the ones who suffer the most. He doesn't know what's happening to him. He's become like a heavyweight child.'

Two of Miguel's sisters are participants in Lopera's Crenuzumab trial. They've been on the drug for nine months. But the results are not due until 2020, and according to Lopera there's been no discernible change to their symptoms. Eager for information, Daniel asked me plainly: based on all the research, what chances did I see for there being a cure in the near future?

I took a moment to consider my answer. Then, head up, I explained how there was more cause for hope now than ever before. Because of families like his, I said, we've learned more in the last ten years than the past one hundred years. I told him how quickly discoveries are made now, and explained why the Colombian community may hold the key to finding the best possible drug. I also said that the next generation of drugs probably wouldn't help his brother but might very well help his children. As for when, I gave him what I considered the most ambitious estimate without being unrealistic: ten years.

He nodded slowly. 'Thank you. Thank you for coming here. To be honest, I don't have money to pay you. But before you leave, you must ride my horse.'

In Colombian author Gabriel García Márquez's multi-generational story of the Buendía family – *One Hundred Years of Solitude*, published in 1967 – he describes the curse of Macondo, a fictional town whose inhabitants are beset by a loss of 'the name and notion of things'. So striking is the condition's likeness to Alzheimer's, one can't help but think the author spent time with the people of Belmira, Yarumal and Angostura, and that he possessed a considerable grasp of the disorder long before the rest of world ever did. Here's just one passage:

When his father told him about his alarm at having forgotten even the most impressive happenings of his childhood, Aureliano explained his method to him, and José Arcadio Buendía put it into practice all through the house and later on imposed it on the whole village. With an inked brush he marked everything with its name: *table, chair, clock, door, wall, bed, pan.* He went to the corral and marked the animals and plants: *cows, goat, pig, hen, cassava, caladium, banana.* Little by little, studying the infinite possibilities of a loss of memory, he realized that the day might come when things would be recognized by their inscriptions but that no one would remember their use. Then he was more explicit. The sign that he hung on the neck of the cow was an exemplary proof of the way in which the inhabitants of Macondo were prepared to fight against loss of memory: *This is the cow. She must be milked every morning so that she will produce milk, and the milk must be boiled in order to be mixed with coffee to make coffee and milk.* Thus they went on living in a reality that was slipping away, momentarily captured by words, but which would escape irremediably when they forgot the values of the written letters.

The inhabitants of Belmira I met were certainly prepared to fight against the loss of memory. And when I left Colombia, I understood something else. That a populace in Iceland, a farmer in India, and a family in Colombia have joined the fight was surely a sign of impending success. The world was closing ranks around Alzheimer's. There was nowhere left for it to hide.

22

Alzheimer's Legacy

Nothing in life is to be feared, it is only to be understood.
Now is the time to understand more, so that we may fear less.

Marie Curie, attributed

'WE'VE BEEN MARRIED fifty-one years. We got married in 1947.' The old man's voice echoed from the speakers in the dimly lit studio. 'The first symptoms were memory loss. She seemed to forget things . . .' He looked down, confused. 'Gradually things got worse and worse . . . I really reached the end of the road, with having to get up in the morning, bathe her, dress her, deciding what clothes she's going to put on, and then of course there are the meals to get ready. But the unfortunate thing is . . .' He paused, voice crumbling, before letting the grief sink in, 'is her not being able to even talk to me . . . It's worse than anything I've come across.'

Professor Nick Fox stopped the video. 'It's a dreadful disease,' he said solemnly, turning to his audience. It was 24 April 2016. I was standing among a crowd of 100 preternaturally quiet Londoners in the Science Museum, watching a clip of one of Fox's patients. It was 8 p.m.; the museum was holding an evening called 'Lost in Thought', a rallying cry for anyone who still hasn't got the memo. Now, on the screen behind Fox, enormous photographs of Alois Alzheimer and Auguste Deter stood like columns, their story enshrined in the monolith of neuroscience.

Fox has been an integral character in my story. It was he, and his protégée Natalie Ryan, both stellar neurologists at London's National Hospital for Neurology and Neurosurgery, who had put me in touch with some of the Alzheimer's families in this book. In addition to seeing patients, Fox now spends considerable time raising public awareness. He recently gave a talk preceding the performance of Nicola Wilson's play *Plaques and Tangles* – portraying the life of a family affected by early-onset dementia – and had, in the past year, released simple online courses that the public could access to learn more about the condition.

'One in three people in this room will get Alzheimer's,' Fox continued. 'One in two will look after someone with Alzheimer's.' He paused and turned again. 'As a society we're sleepwalking into this.'

And so it's time to wake up. We can start by reassessing our priorities. Even though the disease is now heavily ingrained in the public's collective consciousness, Alzheimer's is still woefully under-funded. In the UK alone, the total cost of Alzheimer's is £23 billion a year – more than cancer, heart disease and stroke combined – yet, incredibly, a mere 0.2 per cent of that is actually spent on research. John Trojanowski, a researcher at the University of Pennsylvania, has pointed out that the US spends more money on popcorn, Viagra and anti-ageing creams than Alzheimer's research. This is astounding considering that an additional 7.7 million cases (that we know of) are reported every year. It seems a more horrifying kind of forgetting is taking place in our world. *We* are forgetting them.

If things continue this way, epidemiologists estimate that the total number of Alzheimer's cases will double every twenty years, making dementia the next global pandemic. In that event, the current 46 million patients would represent no more than the tip of a vast, society-crippling iceberg.

So after a century of Alzheimer's research, a journey that's spanned the globe and brought with it a kaleidoscope of blind alleys, high hopes and stark tragedy, the final question is one that's been with us from the very beginning. What is the future for this 'peculiar' disease?

The answer might strike you as somewhat passive, but the hope, for the time being, is to reach where we currently are with diabetes. Diabetes was often a death sentence a century ago, but the advent of molecular biology, and subsequent creation of synthetic human insulin from genetically engineered bacteria, has effectively reduced it to a phantom of its former self. Given how late in life Alzheimer's usually strikes, its own phantom needn't be a phantom for very long. Consider this: if Alzheimer's could be delayed by only one year, there would be 9 million fewer people with the disease by 2050.[1] A five-year delay, some scientists predict, would effectively halve the globe's 46 million sufferers, saving healthcare services approximately $600 billion a year.[2]

So what would this treatment look like? Based on everything we've seen in this book, in the future doctors may not need to administer extensive memory tests or rigorous brain imaging. A drop of blood or a strand of hair might foretell when our minds are set to unravel, and a doctor, with a host of genetically tailored pills to choose from, might know precisely which one to give to ensure lifelong brain health. No longer would we be at the mercy of what is written in our DNA, nor feel compelled to live a spartan existence. We would then be facing some new challenge, safe in the knowledge that memory is untouchable.

In the meantime, here is what we know. We know Alzheimer's is by and large an age-related disorder, but that ageing, in and of itself, is not the root cause. Alzheimer's is, rather, the *product* of processes common in normal ageing. We know that plaques and tangles, for instance, are found in elderly people without causing disease; it's only when they reach a certain threshold that they trigger full-blown dementia. We know that both are necessary – although perhaps not sufficient – to kill neurons, and we know that plaques appear before tangles and are therefore the most attractive target for drug developers.

We know that genetics is central to understanding this disease, and that while only a small minority of people inherit genes for early-onset Alzheimer's – genes such as APP and PSEN1 – many of us possess genetic risk factors that can tip the balance towards dementia, with the APOE4 gene being the strongest risk factor. Undoubtedly, the genetics of the twenty-first century will add a great deal to this story.

But we also know that Alzheimer's is going through a drastic reformation of underlying principles. In the past decade, as methods to conceptualise brain function have advanced, a more holistic understanding of the disease is taking shape. Perhaps the most insightful thesis on this so far – 'The cellular phase of Alzheimer's disease', by Bart De Strooper and Eric Karran in 2016 – argues that the advent of 'systems biology', a method using sophisticated statistics and clever computers, should soon provide the means to generate 'a comprehensive cellular theory of the disorder'.[3] By drawing on individual discoveries from the broad canvas of cell biology, biochemistry, molecular genetics and neuro-imaging, this approach may have the power to piece the entire puzzle together. Just as the Human Connectome Project seeks to map all the neural connections in the brain, systems biology may yield an 'atlas that describes the evolution of Alzheimer's disease', they write.

Detection is another transformative development. Rather than focusing on the ultimate destruction of the brain, our lens has swung 180 degrees, pointing instead at the early, telltale signs of a brain in decline. Even as I write this, a study showing that proteins in human tear fluid might indicate Alzheimer's has reached my desk.[4] Biomarker findings such as these will continue to move the bull's-eye for treatment to middle age, if not younger. And while lifestyle countermeasures have yet to be unanimously approved, we do know that an increasing number of experts are encouraging their use every day. I could probably fill a textbook with all the neurochemical processes we've had to reorganise and reimagine. Alzheimer's research, the scientific field once viewed as a fool's errand, has transmogrified into the grandest of pursuits.

Attitudes still need to change too, of course, for an ageing society can engender as much defeatism as it can defiance. There's an uncomfortable comparison worth mentioning here, which is that cancer, while causing a similar number of deaths each year, receives on average ten times more funding than Alzheimer's. Eliminating cancer is vital, but we shouldn't pour all our efforts into one pandemic only then to be met by another – vanquishing the devil only to meet the deep blue sea. The situation is starker still when comparing Alzheimer's funding to that of HIV/AIDS. In the early 1990s the public lobbied US Congress to allocate 10 per cent of its research budget to help those with the infection. Consequently, it's now a manageable disease and the number of deaths has fallen from 45,000 per year in 1995 to 7,000 in 2013. And yet, the US hasn't readjusted its budget; Alzheimer's receives less funding even though it's now a much bigger problem.[5] This makes no sense. Research funding should reflect disease burden.

On a simpler note, we need more research into the biology of healthy brains. We all marvel at our ability to build cities and skyscrapers, to appreciate art and music, to comprehend planetary motion and organic evolution, to explore the world's oceans and send objects into space, but for all our accomplishments we still don't understand how the organ responsible for such accomplishments works – or why, with time, it breaks down. As the line between Alzheimer's and ageing is further discerned, a better apprehension of the brain's normal inner workings will be crucial to stop the latter spawning the former.

The good news is that people are waking up. In the UK in 2012 former Prime Minister David Cameron launched the 'Dementia Challenge', a government initiative committed to more than doubling research spending on Alzheimer's, from £26.6 million in 2010 to £66.3 million in 2014. In America, Congress has also agreed to boost Alzheimer's funding by 50 per cent, approving a $350 million increase in its 2016 budget. In Europe, private industry is joining public–private schemes such as the European Prevention of Alzheimer's Disease (EPAD) initiative, which aims to create a register of 24,000 people for longitudinal studies and clinical trials. And around the world, big drug companies like Johnson & Johnson, Roche and Novartis are coming back to the table, investing $3.3 billion in research in 2014, according to *Forbes* magazine, more private funding than in any of the preceding ten years.[6] In the end, it all whittles down to money.

Perceptions are also changing. Listening to Fox, I couldn't help noticing the age group of the audience. I'd expected to see mostly middle-aged people, mothers and fathers caring for their elderly parents, perhaps. But these people looked between eighteen and thirty. When I asked some of them why they'd come, it turned out it was for the same reason I decided to write this book: to learn what happened to their grandparents. Fox's campaign was working. A new generation of neurodetectives was here, curious to find the truth.

It was surely this curiosity that provoked a critical moment in not just Alzheimer's but all realms of biology: CRISPR (or Clustered Regularly Interspaced Short Palindromic Repeats) was little more than a repetitive sequence of bacterial DNA when it was first spotted by Japanese scientists in the 1980s. But in 2007 it was discovered that CRISPR is in fact a clever molecular defence system protecting bacteria from viruses: when a virus attacks, CRISPR first stores a fragment of the virus's DNA in the bacterium's genome, recording the threat, and then uses that information to delete any DNA with the same sequence.

Over the past few years, scientists have figured out that CRISPR can also be used as a gene-editing tool for humans. That's because CRISPR is composed of two parts: an enzyme called Cas9, which deletes the viral DNA, and a 'guide' molecule, which ferries Cas9 to the correct location in the genome. By artificially altering the guide molecule, scientists can theoretically add or remove any DNA sequences they want. The technology is in its early days, but the transformative effect it will have on medicine is staggering. Picture it: you go to your doctor and are then referred to a geneticist, who informs you that your son has cystic fibrosis but that they can simply delete the causative gene and replace it with a healthy one. It will be as if he never had the disease. Or you walk into a clinic with an untreatable and inoperable type of cancer, but the geneticist can use CRISPR to edit your immune system's DNA to spot and destroy the malignant cells. And of course, the geneticist could explain that you have the APOE4 gene, that it's a strong risk factor for Alzheimer's, and offer you an APOE2 instead. While discussing that, they could even offer to screen and edit any other genetic risk factors for Alzheimer's as well.

Film enthusiasts will have already drawn parallels to the 1997 film *Gattaca*, a futuristic drama about a world where gene-editing technology has reached its zenith, and, as a consequence, every child has their genome sequenced and edited at birth, ensuring a long and disease-free life. I am not overstating matters when I say that CRISPR is the first inroad towards such a future.

When this day comes, and it will come, there will doubtless be ethical issues concerning designer babies: parents may want to modify genes linked to intelligence, physical strength, behavioural traits, even sexual preference – conceivably leading to another narrative in *Gattaca* in which the technology inadvertently triggers a new form of genetic prejudice and career discrimination, what philosopher Philip Kitcher calls 'laissez-faire eugenics'. It won't be easy to determine where to draw the lines, but as long as we proceed with caution and integrity, that reality should remain unthinkable.

When Fox's speech was over, I wandered through the rest of the exhibit. There were scores of cheerful, energetic researchers showcasing Alzheimer's-themed activities and games for the public. One activity was a giant 'memory wall', on which people had written their most enduring memory. I glanced over some of them. '*Getting engaged in the Sahara desert,'* one person had written. *'Burning my feet on a beach in Greece,'* wrote another. *'Having my hair brushed by my mum whilst looking at a blue car.'*

In a room next door people were playing a retro-style Alzheimer's arcade game, saving virtual brain cells by shooting the killer proteins beta-amyloid and tau. There was a game called 'Operation Alzheimer's', a huge plastic mould of DNA that people had to repair by switching genes on and off. There were stem cell scientists displaying pictures of brains in a dish, physiotherapists discussing the impact of sports and head injuries, neuropsychologists waxing lyrical on Terry Pratchett and visual Alzheimer's. And on and on. Alois Alzheimer would have been stunned.

The most encouraging research right now is the amyloid-based treatments. In August 2016 the US biotech firm Biogen released some early clinical trial results for their new antibody drug, Aducanumab, designed to clear amyloid-beta using the brain's immune cells. For 165 mild Alzheimer's patients, following a year of monthly injections, the drug reduced beta-amyloid levels and slowed cognitive decline. Such news also bodes well for Big Pharma's new BACE inhibitor drugs, designed to stop amyloid accumulating in the first place. The challenge now is to recreate such victories in larger trials. As for the other research areas quickly gathering pace – tangle research, neurogenetics, stem cell technology, young blood, prion biology, off-label cancer drugs, visual Alzheimer's, lifestyle influences – the outlook is good, in that they will either donate key insights to sharpen the blade of amyloid therapeutics, or launch a volley of specialised medications for those who don't respond to such treatment.

I hadn't planned to write a book that involved so many separate strands of thought and areas of research; that ended so open-endedly. The pragmatist in me believed there was only one true path on the road to a cure, and that if I could only find it, I would have the answers I so desperately sought. But now, walking through the exhibit, I suddenly understood why it had to be this way. There was no single path, no one idea to pursue indefinitely. The march of each idea provided the footing for another. And only when enough ideas converge shall we ever reach the summit. As Sir Edmund Hillary once said, it is not the mountain we conquer 'but ourselves'.

Coda

There seems something more speakingly incomprehensible in the powers, the failures, the inequalities of memory, than in any other of our intelligences.

Jane Austen, *Mansfield Park*

IN MARCH 2016 I arranged a final meeting with Carol and Stuart Jennings. They'd taken the familiar trip from Coventry to London for another round of experimental treatment, and kindly set aside some time for me. More than a year had passed since I'd seen Carol. I wasn't quite sure what to expect.

'There's been a slight decline,' Stuart said while the three of us sat in a restaurant near Russell Square. 'Otherwise things have been okay, haven't they, Carol?'

'Hmm yes . . . oh yes,' she replied with characteristic buoyancy. But Carol had undoubtedly slipped. She was quieter, less engaged, more withdrawn. She depended more on Stuart to steady her thoughts. When it was time to order, Stuart led the way while Carol softly echoed fragments of what he said, her mind seemingly taking refuge in his.

I kept remembering something Stuart had said to me when I was at their house. He'd told me that when they were young, as a new couple discovering each other, he rode a clapped-out old motorcycle. I pictured a young Carol sitting on the back, gripping on to Stuart, ready to start their life together. Even now, she was holding on to him, I realised, unaware of her destination but knowing the journey was important. When so much of a person's memory is stripped away, watching their loved ones hold on to and love what's left is a lesson in true intimacy.

'It's her language and conversation that's deteriorated the most.' Stuart lowered his voice several octaves, still uncomfortable speaking of Carol in the third person. 'There are moments of lucidity, where you suddenly realise the person's still there, somewhere . . . But the reality is that when you're with someone for so long, you don't need to communicate. It's been forty years since we met. We know each other so well. There are things which are said but unsaid.'

Said but unsaid. That is the language of Alzheimer's.

'Carol increasingly lives in the present moment,' Stuart continued. 'I myself now live in the present moment. Because living in the moment is the best strategy for a carer. If you keep worrying about tomorrow, you'll wear yourself out.'

Since I'd last spoken to the couple, they'd kept up the fight – attending conferences and staying involved with the London research team (who they now call 'family') – adamantly refusing, as Stuart maintains, to 'go gently into that good night'. As Stuart still works as a university chaplain, he's ensured that somebody now goes to the house every day to check on Carol and her ninety-year-old mother, Joyce. He was telling me about how much more protective he is over Carol, how increasingly aware he is of the limited time she has left, how his life is now about 'squeezing every last drop of her' that he can.

The trial Carol's participating in is a form of immunotherapy, similar to the antibody drugs discussed in chapter six. It might not work. At her stage, it's unlikely to. And she may only be getting a placebo (for the sake of scientific certitude, that information is also hidden from the scientists themselves). But the results no longer matter to the Jennings. 'We're not doing this for ourselves any more,' said Stuart. 'When she was diagnosed, Carol gave me very specific instructions. She'd said, "I want to be involved in research for as long as I possibly can." So now, our struggle is the struggle to take the illness down with us.'

We left the restaurant and walked through the park. Carol was scheduled for another brain scan and I agreed to accompany them as far as the hospital. The day was warm and clear. Elderly men and women reclined on wooden benches while young couples picnicked on the grass. There was a subtle confidence in Carol's stride. Head raised, hands clasped behind her back, she was moving into the final stages with unusual calm. Perhaps the treatment *was* doing something, I mused. Then she looked at me and released a wide smile.

Perhaps indeed.

On a summer day in 2016, sitting alone in his house, Arnold Levi was stirred by the sound of Danie and me, once more waiting patiently at his doorstep. My meeting with Arnold was not to witness his decline – I already knew he wasn't doing well – but to try to catch his final moments of memory and insight, his last tendrils of spirit and inner being.

When I sat beside him and asked how he'd been, he returned a glassy, empty stare. He'd been busy at the film studio, he told me plainly. They needed help with a new production and he was the first person they called. Danie looked at me and gently shook his head. Arnold's mind was now reliving his years as a young man, creating its own reality from residual memories, selecting and magnifying that which brought him the most peace in his life. He looked unnaturally formal, almost paralysed in a state of suspended animation, like a living statue.

While Danie began his usual routine of opening Arnold's mail, I accompanied Arnold to the kitchen to help him make a cup of tea. He watched with a calm, blank look as I reached for a cup and teaspoon. 'Yes . . . yes . . .' he quietly assured me, 'that's what we need . . . isn't it?'

'It says here the doctors want to see you again,' Danie told Arnold as we walked back to the living room.

'Oh,' Arnold responded. 'I wonder what they want to see me about . . .'

'I know you've been taking your medication.'

'Have I? Thank goodness you told me . . . I wouldn't know what I was supposed to be doing . . . You know, I haven't seen you in a *long* time.'

Danie looked at him. 'I saw you two days ago, Arnold.'

'Oh . . . well, did I . . . did I know it?'

I sensed fear in Arnold as he said this. He had the look of a man embroiled in a hopeless inner struggle, his brain searching for connections that no longer existed.

'But why would I have forgotten that?' he implored. 'Is there any idea about that?'

Danie interjected, 'Why don't you show Joseph your photo albums? I'm sure he'd love to see them.' On this bright note, arm-in-arm, Arnold and I headed up to the attic.

'You can put your tea down on that desk,' Arnold instructed, before planting himself on a chair in the corner beneath a small window that blanketed the floor in light. I pulled a large, leather-bound volume off a nearby shelf. The spine crackled as I opened it on Arnold's lap, and he bristled at the sight. The first few pages held pictures of two children clasped in a pretty brunette's arms. 'That's me and my mother and sister,' he whispered with mild confidence. I turned the page to see photographs of a thirty-something, tanned, handsome Arnold in shorts on the beach. He was standing next to Danie's parents – Danie himself, a small boy, nestled among them, grinning at the camera. Hoping to spark a flash of memory, I asked Arnold if he could name the people in the picture. He stared at them for a few seconds and then turned to me. 'I can't give you an answer to this . . .' Then he looked over my shoulder. 'Who's left that tea there?'

It was like watching someone endlessly fall back through time.

My father had attempted this routine with Abbas. In what would become his final trip to visit his ailing father in Iran, he took several old photographs with him – memories of his childhood that he'd kept over the years. As with Arnold, they didn't appear to trigger any signs of reminiscence in Abbas. And yet, I cannot think about that without feeling that we are missing something significant in our apprehension of memory. From one angle, my father's photographs can be seen as mere snapshots of time – moments and experiences – to show Abbas that his past was real, that his life had meaning. From another, they are each an abstraction of the thoughts and feelings that must have occurred in Abbas when he experienced such moments, each a portrait that once hung proudly in the gallery of his mind, each something no amount of brain imaging or cell culturing or gene sequencing will ever recapitulate. When I contemplate my father's act, and every other person no doubt doing the same, I see an attempt to tap into some distant, transient but surviving connection. It is not a futile endeavour. We do it because we know, deep down, a connection is still there.

As a child, I had viewed Abbas's illness as something to fear and something to accept. Alzheimer's was an invisible and terrifying cross to bear, a profound loss that my generation would not see an end to. Now, I understood just how innocent that thinking was. In writing this book I had discovered an astonishingly intricate yet eminently malleable disease. I had witnessed extraordinary minds catapulting neuroscience into unimaginable futures. And I had seen breathtaking acts of human courage and unalloyed sacrifice. We are closer than ever to the abolition of Alzheimer's.

It truly is the beginning of the end.

Resources

The idea is to die young as late as possible.

Ashley Montagu, attributed

W HAT CAN WE do? This is hard to answer, but not impossible. There is advice worth heeding, based on the clinical experience of doctors and nurses. First: early diagnosis is critical. If you are having memory problems that worry you, problems that feel like more than normal ageing, you *must* book an appointment to see your doctor. It truly is a case of the earlier, the better: our methods of detection are rapidly advancing. And while it can be difficult advising someone to seek medical attention for a mental health problem (again I speak from experience: persuading my mother to see a doctor about *anything* is like trying to persuade Kim Jong-un to see a therapist), we must remind people that it is a serious disease.

Second, but no less important: remain active and social for as long as possible. Having family and friends around can have an immensely positive effect on a patient's mood and sense of well-being. In her instructive book *Dementia: The One-Stop Guide*, dementia nurse June Andrews suggests that families should also 'start a private blog, where everyone has their own responsibility to log in and find out for themselves what is going on', and points out that 'friends are not a luxury; they are a necessity for maintaining your health and sanity'. Keeping diaries and calendars and notes will also help manage symptoms. So too, perhaps, will eating well, drinking less alcohol, exercising more, and staying mentally active. A healthy lifestyle might not prevent Alzheimer's, but it may slow it down. On a lighter note, stay positive. Patients often want to keep a sense of humour about what's happening to them, which was certainly true with many of the patients I met.

I am fully persuaded that we will defeat Alzheimer's in our lifetime. In the meantime, perhaps the best advice I can give is to keep looking to the future like the people in this book are – with high spirits, fiery determination and irrepressible optimism.

Some of the best organisations for families, carers and patients:

Age UK
Tel: 0800 678 1174
Email: contact@ageuk.org.uk
Website: www.ageuk.org.uk

Alzheimer's Association
Tel: +1 800 272 3900
Email: info@alz.org
Website: www.alz.org

Alzheimer's Disease Education and Referral Center
Tel: +1 800 438 4380
Email: adear@nia.nih.gov
Website: www.nia.nih.gov/alzheimers

Alzheimer's Disease International
Tel: +44 20 7981 0880
Email: info@alz.co.uk
Website: www.alz.co.uk

Alzheimer's Europe
Tel: +352 29 79 70
Email: info@alzheimer-europe.org
Website: www.alzheimer-europe.org

Alzheimer's Foundation of America

Tel: +1 866 232 8484
Email: info@alzfdn.org
Website: www.alzfdn.org

Alzheimer's Research Forum

Email: contact@alzforum.org
Website: www.alzforum.org

Alzheimer's Research UK

Tel: 0300 111 5555
Email: enquiries@alzheimersresearchuk.org
Website: www.alzheimersresearchuk.org

Alzheimer's Society

Tel: 0300 222 1122
Email: enquiries@alzheimers.org.uk
Website: www.alzheimers.org.uk

Caregiver Action Network

Tel: +1 202 454 3970
Email: info@caregiveraction.org
Website: www.caregiveraction.org

Caregiver.com

Tel: +1 800 829 2734
Email: info@caregiver.com
Website: www.caregiver.com

Carers UK

Tel: 020 7378 4999
Email: info@carersuk.org
Website: www.carersuk.org

Dementia UK

Tel: 0800 888 6678

Email: info@dementiauk.org

Website: www.dementiauk.org

Family Caregiver Alliance

Tel: +1 415 434 3388

Email: info@caregiver.org

Website: www.caregiver.org

National Council for Palliative Care (NCPC)

Tel: 020 7697 1520

Website: www.ncpc.org.uk

NHS Choices

Website: www.nhs.uk

Office of the Public Guardian

Tel: 0870 739 5780

Email: customerservices@publicguardian.gsi.gov.uk

Website: www.gov.uk/government/organisations/office-of-the-public-guardian

Society for Neuroscience

Tel: +1 202 962 4000

Website: www.sfn.org

Acknowledgements

THIS BOOK WAS made possible, first and foremost, by the patients and patient relatives who agreed to be interviewed. I am deeply grateful for their sincerity, openness and astonishing courage. For reasons of anonymity, I shall only cite those who agreed to share their real names; to all the people behind the pseudonyms, I offer you my heartfelt gratitude. I am also enormously thankful to the scientists and physicians for sharing their knowledge and intuition. Their remarkable ability to clarify complex topics provided the animating spirit for my writing, and I hope I have done their work justice.

I'm thankful to Gabriel Aristizábal, Kaj Blennow, Hari Chand, John Collinge, Paige Cramer, Sebastian Crutch, Jeffrey Cummings, Ricardo Dolmetsch, Matteo Farinella, Jens Foell, Nick Fox, Mary Ganguli, Alison Goate, Lawrence Goldstein, John Hardy, Martin Huntley, Victoria Huntley, Sarah Jarvis, Carol Jennings, John Jennings, Stuart Jennings, Mathias Jucker, Sasha Kamb, Ryuta Kawashima, William Klunk, Vijay Kumar, Michael Landon, Gary Landreth, Patrick Lewis, Francisco Lopera, Simon Lovestone, Lucía Madrigal, Karen Magorrian, George Martin, Chester Mathis, Marika Mattsson, Jeremy Mills, Pradeep Narayan, Karoly Nikolich, Thomas Piers, Jeremy Reed, Cressida Robson, Allen Roses, Maria Alejandra Ruiz, Natalie Ryan, Ian Sample, Dale Schenk, Kari Stefánsson, William Summers, Naji Tabet, Rudolph Tanzi, Selina Wray and Henrik Zetterberg.

A special thanks to Carrie Plitt, my exceedingly talented agent at Conville and Walsh, whose comments and revisions made this book significantly better. Additionally, this book could not have been published without the exceptional support of the teams at John Murray and Little, Brown. My wonderful editors, Kate Craigie and Georgina Laycock, provided countless insights in shaping this book.

I owe a huge thanks to Hajra Siraj, my most loyal reader. Her wisdom, guidance and unrivalled compassion helped me on this journey in innumerable ways. Finally, I am for ever indebted to my parents. They sacrificed so much for my education, and taught me at a young age that the purpose of life is to help others.

Notes

Preface: 'A Peculiar Disease'

1. Prince, Comas-Herrera, et al., 'World Alzheimer's Report 2016'.
2. At the time of writing, Alzheimer's overtook heart disease in England and Wales; it is now the leading cause of death. Office for National Statistics, Statistical Bulletin.
3. Reagan, Handwritten letter courtesy of the Ronald Reagan Presidential Foundation and Library.
4. Mukherjee, *The Emperor of All Maladies*, p.39.
5. Lambert, Ibrahim-Verbaas, et al., 'Meta-analysis of 74,046 individuals identifies 11 new susceptibility loci for Alzheimer's disease'.
6. Fraser, Consulting report, July 2015.

Chapter 1: The Psychiatrist with a Microscope

1. World Health Organization (WHO), 'Dementia: Fact Sheet'.
2. Deuteronomy 28:28.
3. Jameson, *Essays on the Changes of the Human Body, at its Different Ages*, p.138.
4. Cicero, *How to Grow Old*, p.77.
5. Galen, *De symptomatum differentiis liber*, in K. Kuhn, *Opera omnia*.
6. Boller, *Handbook of Clinical Neurology* (vol. 89), p.3.
7. Porter, *Madness*, p.42.
8. Hunt, *The Story of Psychology*, p.70.
9. Ibid., p.95.
10. Berrios, *The History of Mental Symptoms*, p.172.
11. Boller, *Handbook of Clinical Neurology* (vol. 89), p.4.

12. Bynum and Porter, *Dictionary of Scientific Quotations*, p.598.
13. Maurer and Maurer, *Alzheimer*, p.55.
14. Ibid., p.84.
15. Ibid., p.152.
16. Ibid., p.163.

Chapter 2: Understanding an Epidemic

1. Newton, 'The identity of Alzheimer's disease and senile dementia and their relationship to senility'.
2. Ballenger, *Self, Senility, and Alzheimer's Disease in Modern America*, p.49.
3. K. B. R. Katzman, *Alzheimer Disease*, p.33.
4. Raine, 'Correspondence: re: Robert Terry and Robert Katzman'.
5. Kidd, 'Paired helical filaments in electron microscopy of Alzheimer's disease'; Terry, Gonatas, Weiss, 'Ultrastructural studies in Alzheimer's presenile dementia'.
6. Ballenger, *Self, Senility, and Alzheimer's Disease in Modern America*, p.81.
7. Roth, Tomlinson, Blessed, 'Correlation between scores for dementia and counts of "senile plaques" in cerebral grey matter of elderly subjects'.
8. Wade, 'Thomas S. Kuhn: Revolutionary Theorist of Science'.
9. R. Katzman, 'Editorial: The prevalence and malignancy of Alzheimer's disease'.

Chapter 3: A Medicine for Memory

1. Reagan, Proclamation 5565 – National Alzheimer's Disease Month.
2. Wolpert, *Malignant Sadness*, p.104.
3. This is a simplification, of course; there is a phenomenon called neuro-plasticity that gives these units a degree of exchangeability. In fact neuroplasticity is why stroke victims can eventually regain certain func-tions, because the brain has literally rewired itself.
4. P. Davies and Maloney, 'Selective loss of central cholinergic neurons in Alzheimer's disease'.
5. Perry, Perry, et al., 'Necropsy evidence of central cholinergic deficits in senile dementia'.
6. Bowen, Smith, et al., 'Neurotransmitter-related enzymes and indices of

hypoxia in senile dementia and other abiotrophies'.

7. B. Taylor, *The Last Asylum*, p.249.
8. Lømo, 'The discovery of long-term potentiation'.
9. Drachman and Leavitt, 'Human memory and the cholinergic system'.
10. Bartus, Dean, et al., 'The cholinergic hypothesis of geriatric memory dysfunction'.
11. Summers, Viesselman, et al., 'Use of THA in treatment of Alzheimer's-like dementia'.
12. Summers, Majovski, et al., 'Oral tetrahydroaminoacridine in long-term treatment of senile dementia, Alzheimer's type'.

Chapter 4: Diagnosis

1. Prince, Wimo, et al., 'World Alzheimer Report 2015'.
2. UK Department of Health, *Dementia*, p.6.
3. Prince, Bryce, Ferri, 'The benefits of early diagnosis and intervention'.

Chapter 5: The Alzheimer's Gene

1. Heston, Mastri, et al., 'Dementia of the Alzheimer type'.
2. Tanzi, *Decoding Darkness*, p.21.
3. Glenner and Wong, 'Alzheimer's disease'.
4. Glenner and Wong, 'Alzheimer's disease and Down's syndrome'.
5. Goldgaber, Lerman, et al., 'Characterization and chromosomal localization of a cDNA encoding brain amyloid of Alzheimer's disease'; Tanzi, Gusella, et al., 'Amyloid beta protein gene'; Robakis, Ramakrishna, et al., 'Molecular cloning and characterization of a cDNA encoding the cerebrovascular and the neuritic plaque amyloid peptides'; Kang, Lemaire, et al., 'The precursor of Alzheimer's disease amyloid A4 protein resembles a cell-surface receptor'.
6. A. Goate, Chartier-Harlin, et al., 'Segregation of a missense mutation in the amyloid precursor protein gene with familial Alzheimer's disease'.
7. Popham, 'Dementia: I have a 50:50 chance'.

Chapter 6: The Science Behind the Headlines

1. This data is for women. In men, heart disease remains the leading cause of death. It's not clear why Alzheimer's is more likely in women; some think it's because women typically live longer, others think genetic differences are responsible.
2. J. A. Hardy and Higgins, 'Alzheimer's disease'.
3. Games, Adams, et al., 'Alzheimer-type neuropathology in transgenic mice overexpressing V717F beta-amyloid precursor protein'.
4. Duff and Hardy, 'Mouse model made'.
5. Saunders, Strittmatter, et al., 'Association of apolipoprotein E allele epsilon 4 with late-onset familial and sporadic Alzheimer's disease'.
6. Roses, 'On the discovery of the genetic association of Apolipoprotein E genotypes and common late-onset Alzheimer disease'.
7. Strittmatter, Saunders, et al., 'Apolipoprotein E'.
8. Small, Ercoli, et al., 'Cerebral metabolic and cognitive decline in persons at genetic risk for Alzheimer's disease'.
9. Herrup, 'The case for rejecting the amyloid cascade hypothesis'.
10. Correspondence with Professor Karoly Nikolich.
11. Shenk, *The Forgetting*, p.68.

Chapter 7: The Second Brain

1. Fields, *The Other Brain*, p.11.
2. McGeer, Itagaki, et al., 'Reactive microglia in patients with senile dementia of the Alzheimer type are positive for the histocompatibility glycoprotein HLA-DR'.
3. M. L. Block and Hong, 'Microglia and inflammation-mediated neuro-degeneration'; M. L. Block, Zecca, Hong, 'Microglia-mediated neurotoxicity'.
4. Jebelli, Hooper, Pocock, 'Microglial p53 activation is detrimental to neuronal synapses during activation-induced inflammation'; Jebelli, Su, et al., 'Glia'; Jebelli, Hooper, Garden, Pocock, 'Emerging roles of p53 in glial cell function in health and disease'.
5. Watkins and Treisman, 'Cognitive impairment in patients with AIDS'.
6. Schenk, 'Amyloid-β immunotherapy for Alzheimer's disease'.

7. Only 18 per cent do, according to one estimate. Arrowsmith, 'Trial watch'.
8. Hock, Konietzko, et al., 'Antibodies against beta-amyloid slow cognitive decline in Alzheimer's disease'.
9. Spinney, 'The forgetting gene'.
10. Klunk, Engler, et al., 'Imaging brain amyloid in Alzheimer's disease with Pittsburgh Compound-B'.
11. Stein, *Four in America*, p.175.

Chapter 8: Swedish Brain Power

1. Arai, Terajima, et al., 'Tau in cerebrospinal fluid'; Blennow and Zetterberg, 'The application of cerebrospinal fluid biomarkers in early diagnosis of Alzheimer disease'.
2. Shahim, Tegner, et al., 'Blood biomarkers for brain injury in concussed professional ice hockey players'; Siman, Shahim, et al., 'Serum SNTF increases in concussed professional ice hockey players and relates to the severity of postconcussion symptoms'.
3. Mapstone, Cheema, et al., 'Plasma phospholipids identify antecedent memory impairment in older adults'.
4. Announced at the US Society for Neuroscience conference, Washington DC, November 2014.
5. Announced at the US Society for Neuroscience conference, San Diego CA, November 2013.
6. Clare Walton, of the Alzheimer's Society, quoted in the *Mail Online*, 13 November 2013.
7. Global AgeWatch Index 2013: Insight report, summary and methodology.
8. Sontag, *Illness as Metaphor*, p.3.

Chapter 9: Stress

1. McEwen and Gianaros, 'Stress- and allostasis-induced brain plasticity'; Marcello, Gardoni, Di Luca, 'Alzheimer's disease and modern lifestyle'.
2. McEwen and Gianaros, 'Central role of the brain in stress and adaptation'.
3. Ganzel, Kim, et al., 'Resilience after 9/11'.

4. Yaffe, Vittinghoff, et al., 'Post-traumatic stress disorder and risk of dementia among U.S. veterans'.

5. Csernansky, Dong, et al., 'Plasma cortisol and progression of dementia in subjects with Alzheimer-type dementia'.

6. Wilson, Barnes, et al., 'Proneness to psychological distress and risk of Alzheimer disease in a biracial community'.

7. Wilson, Arnold, et al., 'Chronic psychological distress and risk of Alzheimer's disease in old age'.

8. Baglietto-Vargas, Chen, et al., 'Short-term modern life-like stress exacerbates Abeta-pathology and synapse loss in 3xTg-AD mice'.

9. Selye, *The Stress of Life*, p.247.

Chapter 10: Diet

1. M. C. Morris, Tangney, et al., 'MIND diet associated with reduced incidence of Alzheimer's disease'.

2. Singh, Parsaik, et al., 'Association of Mediterranean diet with mild cognitive impairment and Alzheimer's disease'.

3. Braniste, Al-Asmakh, et al., 'The gut microbiota influences blood–brain barrier permeability in mice'.

4. Miklossy, 'Alzheimer's disease – a neurospirochetosis'.

5. Frydman-Marom, Levin, et al., 'Orally administrated cinnamon extract reduces β-amyloid oligomerization and corrects cognitive impairment in Alzheimer's disease animal models'.

6. Ngandu, Lehtisalo, et al., 'A 2 year multidomain intervention of diet, exercise, cognitive training, and vascular risk monitoring versus control to prevent cognitive decline in at-risk elderly people (FINGER)'.

Chapter 11: Exercise

1. Nelson, Gard, Tabet, 'Hypertension and inflammation in Alzheimer's disease'.

2. Rockwood, Lindsay, McDowell, 'High blood pressure and dementia'.

3. Nelson and Tabet, 'Slowing the progression of Alzheimer's disease'.

4. Erikson, Voss, et al., 'Exercise training increases size of hippocampus and improves memory'.

5. Farina, Rusted, Tabet, 'The effect of exercise interventions on cognitive outcome in Alzheimer's disease'.

Chapter 12: Brain Training

1. L. Sieg, *Special Report – Can Japan's youth save their ageing nation*, 2001, http://uk.reuters.com/article/uk-japan-youth-idUK-TRE71E1OY20110215
2. Alzheimer's Society, *Brain Training Trial*, 2015, https://www.alzheimers.org.uk/site/scripts/documents_info.php?documentID=3119
3. Mozolic, Hayasaka, Laurienti, 'A cognitive training intervention increases resting cerebral blood flow in healthy older adults'.
4. Wilson, Mendes de Leon, et al., 'Participation in cognitively stimulating activities and risk of incident Alzheimer disease'.
5. Aleman, *Our Ageing Brain*, p.125.
6. Snowdon, *Aging with Grace*, p.118.

Chapter 13: Sleep

1. Moran, Lynch, et al., 'Sleep disturbance in mild to moderate Alzheimer's disease'.
2. J. E. Kang, Lim, et al., 'Amyloid-β dynamics are regulated by orexin and the sleep–wake cycle'.
3. Roh, Huang, et al., 'Disruption of the sleep–wake cycle and diurnal fluctuation of β-amyloid in mice with Alzheimer's disease pathology'.
4. Nedergaard, 'Garbage truck of the brain'.
5. M. P. Walker, '*The Mysteries of Sleep*', https://www.youtube.com/watch?v=rOI45ntOoiA
6. Mander, Marks, et al., 'β-amyloid disrupts human NREM slow waves and related hippocampus-dependent memory consolidation'.
7. Lucey and Holtzman, 'How amyloid, sleep and memory connect'.

Chapter 14: Regeneration

1. Yamanaka, *Lasker Lecture at Albert Einstein College of Medicine*, https://www.youtube.com/watch?v=DQNoyDwCPzM
2. Thomson, Itskovitz-Eldor, et al., 'Embryonic stem cell lines derived from human blastocysts'.
3. Takahashi and Yamanaka, 'Induction of pluripotent stem cells from mouse embryonic and adult fibroblast cultures by defined factors'.
4. Takahashi, Tanabe, et al., 'Induction of pluripotent stem cells from adult human fibroblasts by defined factors'.
5. Van der Worp, Howells, et al., 'Can animal models of disease reliably inform human studies?'.
6. Warren, Tompkins, et al., 'Mice are not men'.
7. Seok, Warren, et al., 'Genomic responses in mouse models poorly mimic human inflammatory diseases'.
8. De Souza, 'Mouse model challenged'.
9. Choi, Kim, et al., 'A three-dimensional human neural cell culture model of Alzheimer's disease'.
10. Hallett, Cooper, et al., 'Long-term health of dopaminergic neuron transplants in Parkinson's disease patients'.
11. Blurton-Jones, Kitazawa, et al., 'Neural stem cells improve cognition via BDNF in a transgenic model of Alzheimer disease'.
12. Mukherjee, *Laws of Medicine (TED)*, p.18.
13. Lapillonne, Kobari, et al., 'Red blood cell generation from human induced pluripotent stem cells'.
14. Tang, Hammack, et al., 'Zika virus infects human cortical neural progenitors and attenuates their growth'.
15. Paul Knoepfler in M. Scudellari, 'How iPS cells changed the world'.

Chapter 15: Young Blood

1. McCay, Pope, et al., 'Parabiosis between old and young rats'.
2. Learoyd, 'The history of blood transfusion prior to the 20th century'.
3. Bert, 'Expériences et considérations sur la greffe animale'.
4. I. M. Conboy, M. J. Conboy, et al., 'Rejuvenation of aged progenitor cells by exposure to a young systemic environment'.

5. Von Radowitz, 'Vampire therapy'.
6. Villeda, Plambeck, et al., 'Young blood reverses age-related impairments in cognitive function and synaptic plasticity in mice'.
7. Villeda, Luo, et al., 'The ageing systemic milieu negatively regulates neurogenesis and cognitive function'.
8. Harrison, Strong, et al., 'Rapamycin fed late in life extends lifespan in genetically heterogeneous mice'.
9. De Grey, *Ending Aging*, p.163.

Chapter 16: Seeds of Dementia

1. Braak and Del Tredici, 'Alzheimer's pathogenesis'.
2. Meyer-Luehmann, Coomaraswamy, et al., 'Exogenous induction of cerebral beta-amyloidogenesis is governed by agent and host'.
3. Lipinski and Hopkins, 'Navigating chemical space for biology and medicine'.
4. Eisele, Obermüller, et al., 'Peripherally applied Abeta-containing inoculates induce cerebral beta-amyloidosis'.
5. R. M. Ridley, Baker, et al., 'Very long term studies of the seeding of beta-amyloidosis in primates'.
6. Jaunmuktane, Mead, et al., 'Evidence for human transmission of amyloid-β pathology and cerebral amyloid angiopathy'.
7. Prusiner, *Madness and Memory*, p.202.
8. To allay fears, the UK's Department of Health created a helpline for anyone who received cadaveric growth hormone and is concerned about their risk of CJD or Alzheimer's.
9. A. Miller, J. Dowd, M. D. Heath, S. M. D. Morris, S. Mosley, P. Nash, . . . R. Williams, *After the storm? UK blood safety and the risk of variant Creutzfeldt-Jakob Disease*, House of Commons Science and Technology Committee, www.publications.parliament.uk/pa/cm201415/cmselect/cmsctech/327/327.pdf
10. Anon., 'Alzheimergate? When miscommunication met sensationalism'.
11. Gye, 'Chief medical officer is accused of trying to discredit impact of controversial study on Alzheimer's before findings were published'.
12. A. Abbott, 'The red-hot debate about transmissible Alzheimer's'.

Chapter 17: Looking but not Seeing

1. Crutch, Lehmann, et al., 'Posterior cortical atrophy'.
2. Pratchett, *Shaking Hands with Death*, p.31.
3. Sacks, *The Mind's Eye*, p.19.
4. Crutch, Schott, et al., 'Shining a light on posterior cortical atrophy'.
5. Whitlock, Sutherland, et al., 'Navigating from hippocampus to parietal cortex'.
6. Breveglieri, Hadjidimitrakis, et al., 'Eye position encoding in three-dimensional space'.

Chapter 18: Between the Devil and the Deep Blue Sea

1. Ariga, 'Common mechanisms of onset of cancer and neurodegenerative diseases'.
2. Staropoli, 'Tumorigenesis and neurodegeneration'.
3. J. Altman, 'Two faces of evil: cancer and neurodegeneration', *Alzforum*, http://www.alzforum.org/news/conference-coverage/two-faces-evil-cancer-and-neurodegeneration
4. Cramer, Cirrito, et al., 'ApoE-directed therapeutics rapidly clear beta-amyloid and reverse deficits in AD mouse models'.
5. Stamps, Bartoshuk, Heilman, 'A brief olfactory test for Alzheimer's disease'.
6. Wang, 'Alzheimer's families clamor for drug'.
7. Pierrot, Lhommel, et al., 'Targretin improves cognitive and biological markers in a patient with Alzheimer's disease'.
8. Shen, 'Studies cast doubt on cancer drug as Alzheimer's treatment'.

Chapter 19: To the Ends of the Earth

1. Salvor Nordal, of the University of Iceland, quoted in E. J. Kirby, 'Iceland's DNA: The world's most precious genes?' BBC, 2014, http://www.bbc.co.uk/news/magazine-27903831
2. Smiley, *The Sagas of the Icelanders*.
3. Jonsson, Atwal, et al., 'A mutation in APP protects against Alzheimer's disease and age-related cognitive decline'.

4. Power, Steinberg, et al., 'Polygenic risk scores for schizophrenia and bipolar disorder predict creativity'.
5. K. W. Burton, 'Anti-Alzheimer's gene may have led to the rise of grandparents', *Science*, http://www.sciencemag.org/news/2015/11/anti-alzheimer-s-gene-may-have-led-rise-grandparents
6. Vassar, 'BACE1 inhibitor drugs in clinical trials for Alzheimer's disease'.
7. Cummings, Morstorf, Zhong, 'Alzheimer's disease drug-development pipeline'.
8. Derek Lowe in M. Burke, 'Why Alzheimer's drugs keep failing', *Scientific American*, https://www.scientificamerican.com/article/why-alzheimer-s-drugs-keep-failing/

Chapter 20: Insights from India

1. Chandra, Ganguli, Ratcliff, et al., 'Studies of the epidemiology of dementia'.
2. Hendrie, Osuntokun, et al., 'Prevalence of Alzheimer's disease and dementia in two communities'.
3. Hendrie, Hall, et al., 'Alzheimer's disease is rare in Cree'.
4. White, Petrovitch, et al., 'Prevalence of dementia in older Japanese-American men in Hawaii'.
5. Ono, Hasegawa, et al., 'Curcumin has potent anti-amyloidogenic effects for Alzheimer's beta-amyloid fibrils in vitro'.
6. F. Yang, Lim, et al., 'Curcumin inhibits formation of amyloid beta oligomers and fibrils, binds plaques, and reduces amyloid in vivo'.
7. Belviranli, Okudan, et al., 'Curcumin improves spatial memory and decreases oxidative damage in aged female rats'.
8. Baum, Lam, et al., 'Six-month randomized, placebo-controlled, double-blind, pilot clinical trial of curcumin in patients with Alzheimer disease'.
9. M. Taylor, Moore, et al., 'Effect of curcumin-associated and lipid ligand-functionalized nanoliposomes on aggregation of the Alzheimer's $A\beta$ peptide'.
10. Popper, *The Logic of Scientific Discovery*, p. 316.

Chapter 21: Clues from Colombia

1. Lemere, Lopera, et al., 'The E280A presenilin 1 Alzheimer mutation produces increased A beta 42 deposition and severe cerebellar pathology'.
2. Sepulveda-Falla, Glatzel, Lopera, 'Phenotypic profile of early-onset familial Alzheimer's disease caused by presenilin-1 E280A mutation'.
3. Belluck, 'Alzheimer's Stalks a Colombian Family'.

Chapter 22: Alzheimer's Legacy

1. Brookmeyer, Johnson, et al., 'Forecasting the global burden of Alzheimer's disease'.
2. Zissimopoulos, Crimmins, St Clair, 'The value of delaying Alzheimer's disease onset'.
3. De Strooper and Karran, 'The cellular phase of Alzheimer's disease'.
4. Kallo, Emri, et al., 'Changes in the chemical barrier composition of tears in Alzheimer's disease reveal potential tear diagnostic biomarkers'.
5. Kaiser, 'What does a disease deserve?'
6. Herper, 'The coming boom in brain medicines'.

Bibliography

Abbott, A., 'The red-hot debate about transmissible Alzheimer's', *Nature*, 531 (7594), 2016, 294–7

Abbott, N. J., Patabendige, A. A., Dolman, D. E., Yusof, S. R., Begley, D. J., 'Structure and function of the blood–brain barrier', *Neurobiology of Disease*, 37 (1), 2010, 13–25

Aguzzi, A., Barres, B. A., Bennett, M. L., 'Microglia: scapegoat, saboteur, or something else?' *Science*, 339 (6116), 2013, 156–61

Aleman, A., *Our Ageing Brain*, Scribe Publications, 2014

Alexander, F. G., and Selesnick, S. T., *The History of Psychiatry*, Harper & Row, 1966

Andrews, J., *Dementia: The One-Stop Guide: Practical Advice for Families, Professionals, and People Living with Dementia and Alzheimer's Disease*, Profile, 2015

Anon., 'Alzheimergate? When miscommunication met sensationalism', *Lancet*, 386 (9999), 2015, 1109

Arai, H., Terajima, M., Miura, M., Higuchi, S., Muramatsu, T., Machida, N., . . . Sasaki, H., 'Tau in cerebrospinal fluid: a potential diagnostic marker in Alzheimer's disease', *Annals of Neurology*, 38 (4), 1995, 649–52

Ariga, H., 'Common mechanisms of onset of cancer and neurodegenerative diseases', *Biological and Pharmaceutical Bulletin* (6), 2015, 795–808

Arrowsmith, J., 'Trial watch: Phase II failures: 2008–2010', *Nature Reviews Drug Discovery*, 10 (5), 2011, 328–9

Baglietto-Vargas, D., Chen, Y., Suh, D., Ager, R. R., Rodriguez-Ortiz, C. J., Medeiros, R., . . . LaFerla, F. M., 'Short-term modern life-like stress exacerbates Abeta-pathology and synapse loss in 3xTg-AD mice', *Journal of Neurochemistry*, 134 (5), 2015, 915–26

Ballatore, C., Lee, V. M., Trojanowski, J. Q., 'Tau-mediated neurodegeneration in Alzheimer's disease and related disorders', *Nature Reviews Neuroscience*, 8 (9), 2007, 663–72

Ballenger, J. F., *Self, Senility, and Alzheimer's Disease in Modern America: A History*, Johns Hopkins University Press, 2006

Bartus, R. T., Dean, R. L., 3rd, Beer, B., Lippa, A. S., 'The cholinergic hypothesis of geriatric memory dysfunction', *Science*, 217 (4558), 1982, 408–14

Baum, L., Lam, C. W., Cheung, S. K., Kwok, T., Lui, V., Tsoh, J., 'Six-month randomized, placebo-controlled, double-blind, pilot clinical trial of curcumin in patients with Alzheimer disease', *Journal of Clinical Psychopharmacology*, 28 (1), 2008, 110–13

Becker, A. J., McCulloch, E. A., Till, J. E., 'Cytological demonstration of the clonal nature of spleen colonies derived from transplanted mouse marrow cells', *Nature*, 197, 1963, 452–4

Belluck, P., 'Alzheimer's Stalks a Colombian Family', *New York Times*, 1 June 2010

Belviranli, M., Okudan, N., Atalik, K., Öz, M., 'Curcumin improves spatial memory and decreases oxidative damage in aged female rats', *Biogerontology*, 14 (2), 2013, 187–96

Berrios, G., *The History of Mental Symptoms: Descriptive Psychopathology Since the Nineteenth Century*, Cambridge University Press, 1996

Bert, P., 'Expériences et considérations sur la greffe animale', *Journal de L'Anatomie et de la Physiologie* . . . 1, 1864, 69–87

Bessis, A., Bechade, C., Bernard, D., Roumier, A., 'Microglial control of neuronal death and synaptic properties', *Glia*, 55 (3), 2007, 233–8

Bianconi, E., Piovesan, A., Facchin, F., Beraudi, A., Casadei, R., Frabetti, F., . . . Canaider, S., 'An estimation of the number of cells in the human body', *Annals of Human Biology*, 40 (6), 2013, 463–71

Bishop, N. A., Lu, T., Yankner, B. A., 'Neural mechanisms of ageing and cognitive decline', *Nature*, 464 (7288), 2010, 529–35

Blennow, K., and Zetterberg, H., 'The application of cerebrospinal fluid biomarkers in early diagnosis of Alzheimer disease', *Medical Clinics of North America*, 97 (3), 2013, 369–76

Blennow, K., Zetterberg, H., Fagan, A. M., 'Fluid biomarkers in Alzheimer disease', *Cold Spring Harbour Perspectives in Medicine*, 2 (9), 2012, a006221

Block, M. L., and Hong, J. S., 'Microglia and inflammation-mediated neurodegeneration: multiple triggers with a common mechanism', *Progress in Neurobiology*, 76 (2), 2005, 77–98

Block, M. L., Zecca, L., Hong, J. S., 'Microglia-mediated neurotoxicity: uncovering the molecular mechanisms', *Nature Reviews Neuroscience*, 8 (1), 2007, 57–69

Block, S., *The Story of Forgetting*, Faber & Faber, 2009

Blurton-Jones, M., Kitazawa, M., Martinez-Coria, H., Castello, N. A., Müller, J. F. Loring, J. F., . . . LaFerla, F. M., 'Neural stem cells improve cognition via BDNF in a transgenic model of Alzheimer disease', *Proceedings of the National Academy of Sciences of the United States of America*, 106 (32), 2009, 13594–9

Boller, F., *Handbook of Clinical Neurology*, vol. 89, Chapter 1: History of Dementia, Elsevier, 2008

Bowen, D. M., Smith, C. B., White, P., Davison, A. N., 'Neurotransmitter-related enzymes and indices of hypoxia in senile dementia and other abiotrophies', *Brain*, 99 (3), 1976, 459–96

Braak, H., and Del Tredici, K., 'Alzheimer's pathogenesis: is there neuron-to-neuron propagation?', *Acta Neuropathologica*, 121 (5), 2011, 589–95

Bradl, M., and Lassmann, H., 'Oligodendrocytes: biology and pathology', *Acta Neuropathologica*, 119 (1), 2010, 37–53

Braniste, V., Al-Asmakh, M., Kowa, C., Anuar, F., Abbaspour, A., Toth, M., . . . Pettersson, S., 'The gut microbiota influences blood–brain barrier permeability in mice', *Science Translational Medicine*, 6 (263), 2014, 263ra158

Bray, D., *Wetware: A Computer in Every Living Cell*, Yale University Press, 2011

Breveglieri, R., Hadjidimitrakis, K., Bosco, A., Sabatini, S. P., Galletti, C., Fattori, P., 'Eye position encoding in three-dimensional space: integration of version and vergence signals in the medial posterior parietal cortex', *Journal of Neuroscience*, 32 (1), 2012, 159–69

Brookmeyer, R., Johnson, E., Ziegler-Graham, K., Arrighi, H. M., 'Forecasting the global burden of Alzheimer's disease', *Alzheimer's & Dementia*, 3 (3), 2007, 186–91

Brown, G. C., 'Nitric oxide and neuronal death', *Nitric Oxide*, 23 (3), 2010, 153–65

Brown, G. C., and Neher, J. J., 'Inflammatory neurodegeneration and mechanisms of microglial killing of neurons', *Molecular Neurobiology*, 41 (2–3), 2010, 242–7

Brundin, P., Melki, R., Kopito, R., 'Prion-like transmission of protein aggregates in neurodegenerative diseases', *Nature Reviews Molecular Cell Biology*, 11 (4), 2010, 301–7

Bynum, W. F., and Porter, R, *Dictionary of Scientific Quotations*, Oxford University Press, 2006

Callaway, E., 'Alzheimer's drugs take a new tack', *Nature*, 489 (7414), 2012, 13–14

Caraci, F., Copani, A., Nicoletti, F., Drago, F., 'Depression and Alzheimer's disease: neurobiological links and common pharmacological targets', *European Journal of Pharmacology*, 626 (1), 2010, 64–71

Carey, N., *The Epigenetics Revolution: How Modern Biology is Rewriting Our Understanding of Genetics, Disease and Inheritance*, Columbia University Press, 2012

Carper, J., *100 Simple Things You Can Do To Prevent Alzheimer's and Age-Related Memory Loss*, Vermilion, 2011

Catindig, J. A., Venketasubramanian, N., Ikram, M. K., Chen, C., 'Epidemiology of dementia in Asia: insights on prevalence, trends and novel risk factors', *Journal of Neurological Sciences*, 321 (1–2), 2012, 11–16

Chandra, V., DeKosky, S. T., Pandav, R., Johnston, J., Belle, S. H., Ratcliff, G., Ganguli, M., 'Neurologic factors associated with cognitive impairment in a rural elderly population in India: the Indo–US Cross-National Dementia Epidemiology Study', *Journal of Geriatric Psychiatry and Neurology*, 11 (1), 1998, 11–17

Chandra, V., Ganguli, M., Pandav, R., Johnston, J., Belle, S., DeKosky, S. T., 'Prevalence of Alzheimer's disease and other dementias in rural India: the Indo–US Study', *Neurology*, 51 (4), 1998, 1000–8

Chandra, V., Ganguli, M., Ratcliff, G., Pandav, R., Sharma, S., Belle, S., . . . Nath, L., 'Practical issues in cognitive screening of elderly illiterate populations in developing countries. The Indo–US Cross-National Dementia Epidemiology Study', *Aging Clinical and Experimental Research*, 10 (5), 1998, 349–57

Chandra, V., Ganguli, M., Ratcliff, G., Pandav, R., Sharma, S., Gilby, J., . . . Nath, L., 'Studies of the epidemiology of dementia: comparisons between developed and developing countries', *Aging Clinical and Experimental Research*, 6 (5), 1994, 307–21

Chandra, V., Pandav, R., Dodge, H. H., Johnston, J. M., Belle, S. H., DeKosky, S. T., Ganguli, M., 'Incidence of Alzheimer's disease in a rural community in India: the Indo–US Study', *Neurology*, 57 (6), 2001, 985–9

Choi, S. H., Kim, Y. H., Hebisch, M., Sliwinski, C., Lee, S., D'Avanzo, C., . . . Kim, D. Y., 'A three-dimensional human neural cell culture model of Alzheimer's disease', *Nature*, 515 (7526), 2014, 274–8.

Cicero, M. T., *How to Grow Old: Ancient Wisdom for the Second Half of Life*, Princeton University Press, 2016

Clare, R., King, V. G., Wirenfeldt, M., Vinters, H. V., 'Synapse loss in dementias', *Journal of Neuroscience Research*, 88 (10), 2010, 2083–90

Cohen, A. D., and Klunk, W. E., 'Early detection of Alzheimer's disease using PiB and FDG PET', *Neurobiology of Disease*, 72 Pt A, 2014, 117–22

Conboy, I. M., Conboy, M. J., Wagers, A. J., Girma, E. R., Weissman, I. L., Rando, T. A., 'Rejuvenation of aged progenitor cells by exposure to a young systemic environment', *Nature*, 433 (7027), 2005, 760–4

Conboy, M. J., Conboy, I. M., Rando, T. A., 'Heterochronic parabiosis: historical perspective and methodological considerations for studies of aging and longevity', *Aging Cell*, 12 (3), 2013, 525–30

Corcoran, D., *The New York Times Book of Science: More Than 100 Years of Groundbreaking Scientific Coverage*, Sterling, 2015

Cramer, P. E., Cirrito, J. R., Wesson, D. W., Lee, C. Y., Karlo, J. C., Zinn, A. E., . . . Landreth, G. E., 'ApoE-directed therapeutics rapidly clear beta-amyloid and reverse deficits in AD mouse models', *Science*, 335 (6075), 2012, 1503–6

Crutch, S. J., Lehmann, M., Schott, J. M., Rabinovici, G. D., Rossor, M. N., Fox, N. C., 'Posterior cortical atrophy', *Lancet Neurology*, 11 (2), 2012, 170–8

Crutch, S. J., Schott, J. M., Rabinovici, G. D., Boeve, B. F., Cappa, S. F., Dickerson, B. C., . . . Fox, N. C., 'Shining a light on posterior cortical atrophy', *Alzheimer's & Dementia*, 9 (4), 2013, 463–5

Csernansky, J. G., Dong, H., Fagan, A. M., Wang, L., Xiong, C., Holtzman, D. M., Morris, J. C., 'Plasma cortisol and progression of dementia in subjects with Alzheimer-type dementia', *American Journal of Psychiatry*, 163 (12), 2006, 2164–9

Cummings, J. L., Morstorf, T., Zhong, K., 'Alzheimer's disease drug-development pipeline: few candidates, frequent failures', *Alzheimer's Research and Therapy*, 6 (4), 2014, 37

Davies, J. A., *Life Unfolding: How the Human Body Creates Itself*, Oxford University Press, 2015

Davies, P., and Maloney, A. J., 'Selective loss of central cholinergic neurons in Alzheimer's disease', *Lancet*, 2 (8000), 1976, 1403

Dawkins, R., *The Selfish Gene: 40th Anniversary Edition*, Oxford University Press, 2016

De Grey, A., *Ending Aging: The Rejuvenation Breakthroughs That Could Reverse Human Aging in Our Lifetime*, St Martin's Griffin, 2008

De Souza, N., 'Mouse model challenged', *Nature Methods*, 10 (4), 2013, 288

De Strooper, B., and Karran, E., 'The cellular phase of Alzheimer's disease', *Cell*, 164 (4), 2016, 603–15

Di Luca, M., and Olesen, J., 'The cost of brain diseases: a burden or a challenge?', *Neuron*, 82 (6), 2014, 1205–8

Drachman, D. A., and Leavitt, J., 'Human memory and the cholinergic system. A relationship to aging?', *Archives of Neurology*, 30 (2), 1974, 113–21

Drake, A. C., 'Of mice and men: what rodent models don't tell us', *Cellular & Molecular Immunology*, 10 (4), 2013, 284–5

Duff, K., and Hardy, J., 'Mouse model made', *Nature*, 373 (6514), 1995, 476–7

Eisele, Y. S., Obermüller, U., Heilbronner, G., Baumann, F., Kaeser, S. A., Wolburg, H., . . . Jucker, M., 'Peripherally applied Abeta-containing inoculates induce cerebral beta-amyloidosis', *Science*, 330 (6006), 2010, 980–2

Enders, G., *Gut*, Scribe Publications, 2015

Erikson, K. I., Voss, M. W., Prakash, R. S., Basak, C., Szabo, A., Chaddock, L., . . . Kramer, A. F., 'Exercise training increases size of hippocampus and improves memory', *Proceedings of the National Academy of Sciences of the United States of America*, 108 (7), 2011, 3017–22

Eroglu, C., and Barres, B. A., 'Regulation of synaptic connectivity by glia', *Nature*, 468 (7321), 2010, 223–31

Farina, N., Rusted, J., Tabet, N., 'The effect of exercise interventions on cognitive outcome in Alzheimer's disease: a systematic review', *International Psychogeriatrics*, 26 (1), 2014, 9–18

Farrer, L. A., 'Expanding the genomic roadmap of Alzheimer's disease', *Lancet Neurology*, 14 (8), 2015, 783–5

Ferry, J. S. G., *The Common Thread*, Corgi, 2009

Fields, R. D., *The Other Brain: The Scientific and Medical Breakthroughs That Will Heal Our Brains and Revolutionize Our Health*, Simon & Schuster, 2011

Fillenbaum, G. G., Chandra, V., Ganguli, M., Pandav, R., Gilby, J. E., Seaberg, E. C., . . . Nath, L. M., 'Development of an activities of daily living scale to screen for dementia in an illiterate rural older population in India', *Age and Ageing*, 28 (2), 1999, 161–8

Finger, S., *Origins of Neuroscience: A History of Explorations into Brain Function*, Oxford University Press, 2001

Fraser, L., Consulting report, 'Estimation of future cases of dementia from those born in 2015', Alzheimer's Research UK and Office of Health Economics, 17 July 2015

Frisoni, G. B., and Visser, P. J., 'Biomarkers for Alzheimer's disease: a controversial topic', *Lancet Neurology*, 14 (8), 2015, 781–3

Frydman-Marom, A., Levin, A., Farfara, D., Benromano, T., Scherzer-Attali, R., Peled, S., . . . Ovadia, M., 'Orally administered cinnamon extract reduces β-amyloid oligomerization and corrects cognitive impairment in Alzheimer's disease animal models', *PloS One*, 6 (1), 2011, e16564

Galen, C., *De symptomatum differentiis liber*, trans. in K. Kuhn, *Opera omnia* (vol. 7), Leipzig: Knobloch, 1821–33

Games, D., Adams, D., Alessandrini, R., Barbour, R., Berthelette, P., Blackwell, C., . . . Zhao, J., 'Alzheimer-type neuropathology in transgenic mice overexpressing V717F beta-amyloid precursor protein', *Nature*, 373 (6514), 1995, 523–7

Gandy, S., and Heppner, F. L., 'Microglia as dynamic and essential components of the amyloid hypothesis', *Neuron*, 78 (4), 2013, 575–7

Ganguli, M., Chandra, V., Gilby, J. E., Ratcliff, G., Sharma, S. D., Pandav, R., . . . Belle, S., 'Cognitive test performance in a community-based nondemented elderly sample in rural India: the Indo-US Cross-National Dementia Epidemiology Study', *International Psychogeriatrics*, 8 (4), 1996, 507–24

Ganguli, M., Chandra, V., Kamboh, M. I., Johnston, J. M., Dodge, H. H., Thelma, B. K., . . . DeKosky, S. T., 'Apolipoprotein E polymorphism and Alzheimer disease: the Indo-US Cross-National Dementia Study', *Archives of Neurology*, 57 (6), 2000, 824–30

Ganguli, M., Dube, S., Johnston, J. M., Pandav, R., Chandra, V., Dodge, H. H., 'Depressive symptoms, cognitive impairment and functional impairment in a rural elderly population in India: a Hindi version of the geriatric depression scale (GDS-H)', *International Journal of Geriatric Psychiatry*, 14 (10), 1999, 807–20

Ganguli, M., Ratcliff, G., Chandra, V., Sharma, S., Gilby, J., Pandav, R., . . . Dekosky, S., 'A Hindi version of the MMSE: the development of a cognitive screening instrument for a largely illiterate rural elderly population in India', *International Journal of Geriatric Psychiatry*, 10 (5), 1994, 367–77

Ganzel, B. L., Kim, P., Glover, G. H., Temple, E., 'Resilience after 9/11: multimodal neuroimaging evidence for stress-related change in the healthy adult brain', *NeuroImage*, 40 (2), 2008, 788–95

Garden, G. A., and La Spada, A. R., 'Intercellular (mis)communication in neurodegenerative disease', *Neuron*, 73 (5), 2012, 886–901

Garden, G. A., and Moller, T., 'Microglia biology in health and disease', *Journal of Neuroimmune Pharmacology*, 1 (2), 2006, 127–37

Genova, L., *Still Alice*, Simon & Schuster, 2015

Glass, C. K., Saijo, K., Winner, B., Marchetto, M. C., Gage, F. H., 'Mechanisms underlying inflammation in neurodegeneration', *Cell*, 140 (6), 2010, 918–34

Glenner, G. G., and Wong, C. W., 'Alzheimer's disease: initial report of the purification and characterization of a novel cerebrovascular amyloid protein', *Biochemical and Biophysical Research Communications*, 120 (3), 1984, 885–90

——, 'Alzheimer's disease and Down's syndrome: sharing of a unique cerebrovascular amyloid fibril protein', *Biochemical and Biophysical Research Communications*, 122 (3), 1984, 1131–5

Goate, A., Chartier-Harlin, M., Mullan, M., Brown, J., Crawford, F., Fidani, L., . . . Hardy, J., 'Segregation of a missense mutation in the amyloid precursor protein gene with familial Alzheimer's disease', *Nature*, 349 (6311), 1991, 704–6

Goate, A. M., Owen, M. J., James, L. A., Mullan, M. J., Rossor, M. N., Haynes, A. R., . . . Hardy, J. A., 'Predisposing locus for Alzheimer's disease on chromosome 21', *Lancet*, 1 (8634), 1989, 352–5

Goedert, M., Wischik, C. M., Crowther, R. A., Walker, J. E., Klug, A., 'Cloning and sequencing of the cDNA encoding a core protein of the paired helical filament of Alzheimer disease: identification as the microtubule-associated protein tau', *Proceedings of the National Academy of Sciences of the United States of America*, 85 (11), 1988, 4051–5

Goldgaber, D., Lerman, M., McBride, O. W., Saffiotti, U., Gajdusek, D. C., 'Characterization and chromosomal localization of a cDNA encoding brain amyloid of Alzheimer's disease', *Science*, 235 (4791), 1987, 877–80

Greenberg, S. M., Bacskai, B. J., Hyman, B. T., 'Alzheimer disease's double-edged vaccine', *Nature Medicine*, 9 (4), 2003, 389–90

Gye, H., 'Chief medical officer is accused of trying to discredit impact of controversial study on Alzheimer's before findings were published', *Mail Online*, 24 September 2015

Hallett, P. J., Cooper, O., Sadi, D., Robertson, H., Mendez, I., Isacson, O., 'Long-term health of dopaminergic neuron transplants in Parkinson's disease patients', *Cell Reports*, 7 (6), 2014, 1755–61

Hampel, H., Frank, R., Broich, K., Teipel, S. J., Katz, R. G., Hardy, J., . . . Blennow, K., 'Biomarkers for Alzheimer's disease: academic, industry and regulatory perspectives', *Nature Reviews Drug Discovery*, 9 (7), 2010, 560–74

Hardy, J., 'A hundred years of Alzheimer's disease research', *Neuron*, 52 (1), 2006, 3–13

Hardy J., and Selkoe, D. J., 'The amyloid hypothesis of Alzheimer's disease: progress and problems on the road to therapeutics', *Science*, 297 (5580), 2002, 353–6

Hardy, J. A., and Higgins, G. A., 'Alzheimer's disease: the amyloid cascade hypothesis', *Science*, 256 (5054), 1992, 184–5

Harrison, D. E., Strong, R., Sharp, Z. D., Nelson, J. F., Astle, C. M., Flurkey, K., 'Rapamycin fed late in life extends lifespan in genetically hetero-geneous mice', *Nature*, 460 (7253), 2009, 392–5

Hauser, P. S., and Ryan, R. O., 'Impact of apolipoprotein E on Alzheimer's disease', *Current Alzheimer Research*, 10 (8), 2013, 809–17

Hendrie, H. C., Hall, K. S., Pillay, N., Rodgers, D., Prince, C., Norton, J., . . . Osuntokun, B., 'Alzheimer's disease is rare in Cree', *International Psychogeriatrics*, 5 (1), 1993, 5–14

Hendrie, H. C., Osuntokun, B., Hall, K. S., Ogunniyi, A. O., Hui, S. L., Unverzagt, F. W., . . . Musick, B. S., 'Prevalence of Alzheimer's disease and dementia in two communities: Nigerian Africans and African Americans', *American Journal of Psychiatry*, 152 (10), 1995, 1485–92

Heppner, F. L., Ransohoff, R. M., Becher, B., 'Immune attack: the role of inflammation in Alzheimer disease', *Nature Reviews Neuroscience*, 16 (6), 2015, 358–72

Herper, M., 'The coming boom in brain medicines', *Forbes*, 2 March 2015

Herrup, K., 'The case for rejecting the amyloid cascade hypothesis', *Nature Neuroscience*, 18 (6), 2015, 794–9

Heston, L. L., Mastri, A. R., Anderson, V. E., White, J., 'Dementia of the Alzheimer type. Clinical genetics, natural history, and associated condi-tions', *Archives of General Psychiatry*, 38 (10), 1981, 1085–90

Hock, C., Konietzko, U., Streffer, J. R., Tracy, J., Signorell, A., Müller-Tillmanns, B., . . . Nitsch, R. M., 'Antibodies against beta-amyloid slow cognitive decline in Alzheimer's disease', *Neuron*, 38 (4), 2003, 547–54

Humpel, C., 'Identifying and validating biomarkers for Alzheimer's disease', *Trends in Biotechnology*, 29 (1), 2011, 26–32

Hunsberger, J. G., Rao, M., Kurtzberg, J., Bulte, J. W. M., Atala, A., LaFerla, F. M., . . . Doraiswamy, P. M., 'Accelerating stem cell trials for Alzheimer's disease', *Lancet Neurology*, 15 (2), 2016, 219–30

Hunt, M., *The Story of Psychology*, Anchor Books, 2007

Inoue, H., Nagata, N., Kurokawa, H., Yamanaka, S., 'iPS cells: a game changer for future medicine', *EMBO J*, 33 (5), 2014, 409–17

Israel, M. A., Yuan, S. H., Bardy, C., Reyna, S. M., Mu, Y., Herrera, C., . . . Goldstein, L. S., 'Probing sporadic and familial Alzheimer's disease using induced pluripotent stem cells', *Nature*, 482 (7384), 2012, 216–20

Jameson, T., *Essays on the Changes of the Human Body, at its Different Ages*, Nabu Press, 2011

Jaunmuktane, Z., Mead, S., Ellis, M., Wadsworth, J. D., Nicoll, A. J., Kenny, J., . . . Brandner, S., 'Evidence for human transmission of amyloid-β pathology and cerebral amyloid angiopathy', *Nature*, 525 (7568), 2015, 247–50

Jebelli, J., Hooper, C., Pocock, J. M., 'Microglial p53 activation is detrimental to neuronal synapses during activation-induced inflammation: implications for neurodegeneration', *Neuroscience Letters*, 583, 2014, 92–7

Jebelli, J. D., Hooper, C., Garden, G. A., Pocock, J. M., 'Emerging roles of p53 in glial cell function in health and disease', *Glia*, 60 (4), 2012, 515–25

Jebelli, J., Su, W., Hopkins, S., Pocock, J., Garden, G. A., 'Glia: guardians, gluttons, or guides for the maintenance of neuronal connectivity?', *Annals of the New York Academy of Sciences*, 1351, 2015, 1–10

Jones, S., *The Language of the Genes*, Flamingo, 2000

Jonsson, T., Atwal, J. K., Steinberg, S., Snaedal, J., Jonsson, P. V., Bjornsson, S., . . . Stefansson, K., 'A mutation in APP protects against Alzheimer's disease and age-related cognitive decline', *Nature*, 488 (7409), 2012, 96–9

Justice, N. J., Huang, L., Tian, J. B., Cole, A., Pruski, M., Hunt, A. J., Jr., . . . Zheng, H., 'Posttraumatic stress disorder-like induction elevates beta-amyloid levels, which directly activates corticotropin-releasing factor neurons to exacerbate stress responses', *Journal of Neuroscience*, 35 (6), 2015, 2612–23

Kaiser, J., '"Rejuvenation factor" in blood turns back the clock in old mice', *Science*, 344 (6184), 2014, 570–1

——, 'What does a disease deserve?', *Science*, 350 (6263), 2015, 900–2

Kallo, G., Emri, M., Varga, Z., Ujhelyi, B., Tozser, J., Csutak, A., Csosz, E., 'Changes in the chemical barrier composition of tears in Alzheimer's disease reveal potential tear diagnostic biomarkers', *PLoS One*, 11 (6), 2016, e0158000

Kandel, E. R., Schwartz, J. H., Jessell, T. M., Siegelbaum, S. A., Hudspeth, A. J., *Principles of Neural Science, Fifth Edition*, McGraw-Hill Education/Medical, 2012

Kaneko, M., Sano, K., Nakayama, J., Amano, N., 'Nasu-Hakola disease: the first case reported by Nasu and review: the 50th anniversary of Japanese Society of Neuropathology', *Neuropathology*, 30 (5), 2010, 463–70

Kang, J., Lemaire, H. G., Unterbeck, A., Salbaum, J. M., Masters, C. L., Grzeschik, K. H., . . . Müller-Hill, B., 'The precursor of Alzheimer's disease amyloid A4 protein resembles a cell-surface receptor', *Nature*, 325 (6106), 1987, 733–6

Kang, J. E., Lim, M. M., Bateman, R. J., Lee, J. J., Smyth, L. P., Cirrito, J. R., . . . Holtzman, D. M., 'Amyloid-β dynamics are regulated by orexin and the sleep–wake cycle', *Science*, 326 (5955), 2009, 1005–7

Katsimpardi, L., Litterman, N. K., Schein, P. A., Miller, C. M., Loffredo, F. S., Wojtkiewicz, G. R., . . . Rubin, L. L., 'Vascular and neurogenic rejuvenation of the aging mouse brain by young systemic factors', *Science*, 344 (6184), 2014, 630–4

Katzman, K. B. R., *Alzheimer Disease: The Changing View*, Academic Press, 2000

Katzman, R., 'Editorial: the prevalence and malignancy of Alzheimer disease. A major killer', *Archives of Neurology*, 33 (4), 1976, 217–18

Kean, S., *The Tale of the Duelling Neurosurgeons: The History of the Human Brain as Revealed by True Stories of Trauma, Madness, and Recovery*, Black Swan, 2015

Kidd, M., 'Paired helical filaments in electron microscopy of Alzheimer's disease', *Nature*, 197, 1963, 192–3

Kim, J., and Holtzman, D. M., 'Prion-like behavior of amyloid-β', *Science*, 330 (6006), 2010, 918–19

Klunk, W. E., Engler, H., Nordberg, A., Wang, Y., Blomqvist, G., Holt, D. P., . . . Långström, B., 'Imaging brain amyloid in Alzheimer's disease with Pittsburgh Compound-B', *Annals of Neurology*, 55 (3), 2004, 306–19

Kondo, T., Asai, M., Tsukita, K., Kutoku, Y., Ohsawa, Y., Sunada, Y., . . . Inoue, H., 'Modeling Alzheimer's disease with iPSCs reveals stress phenotypes associated with intracellular Abeta and differential drug responsiveness', *Cell Stem Cell*, 12 (4), 2013, 487–96

Kuhn, T. S., *The Structure of Scientific Revolutions*, University of Chicago Press, 2012

Lambert, J. C., Ibrahim-Verbaas, C. A., Harold, D., Naj, A. C., Sims, R., Bellenguez, C., . . . Amouyel, P., 'Meta-analysis of 74,046 individuals identifies 11 new susceptibility loci for Alzheimer's disease', *Nature Genetics*, 45 (12), 2013, 1452–8

Lane, N., *Power, Sex, Suicide: Mitochondria and the Meaning of Life*, Oxford University Press, 2006

Lapillonne, H., Kobari, L., Mazurier, C., Tropel, P., Giarratana, M. C., Zanella-Cleon, I., . . . Douay, L., 'Red blood cell generation from human induced pluripotent stem cells: perspectives for transfusion medicine', *Haematologica*, 95 (10), 2010, 1651–9

Learoyd, P., 'The history of blood transfusion prior to the 20th century', *Transfusion Medicine*, 22 (5), 2012, 308–14

LeDoux, J., *Synaptic Self: How Our Brains Become Who We Are*, Penguin, 2003

Lee, M., Bard, F., Johnson-Wood, K., Lee, C., Hu, K., Griffith, S. G., . . . Seubert, P., 'Abeta42 immunization in Alzheimer's disease generates Abeta N-terminal antibodies', *Annals of Neurology*, 58 (3), 2005, 430–5

Leff, J., 'Science and society: the psychiatric revolution: care in the community', *Nature Reviews Neuroscience*, 3 (10), 2002, 821–4

Lemere, C. A., Lopera, F., Kosik, K. S., Lendon, C. L., Ossa, J., Saido, T. C., . . . Arango, J. C., 'The E280A presenilin 1 Alzheimer mutation produces increased A beta 42 deposition and severe cerebellar pathology', *Nature Medicine*, 2 (10), 1996, 1146–50

Levy-Lahad, E., Wasco, W., Poorkaj, P., Romano, D. M., Oshima, J., Pettingell, W. H., . . . Tanzi, R. E., 'Candidate gene for the chromosome 1 familial Alzheimer's disease locus', *Science*, 269 (5226), 1995, 973–7

Levy-Lahad, E., Wijsman, E. M., Nemens, E., Anderson, L., Goddard, K. A., Weber, J. L., . . . Schellenberg, G. D., 'A familial Alzheimer's disease locus on chromosome 1', *Science*, 269 (5226), 1995, 970–3

Lipinski, C., and Hopkins, A., 'Navigating chemical space for biology and medicine', *Nature*, 432 (7019), 2004, 855–61

Loffredo, F. S., Steinhauser, M. L., Jay, S. M., Gannon, J., Pancoast, J. R., Yalamanchi, P., . . . Lee, R. T., 'Growth differentiation factor 11 is a circulating factor that reverses age-related cardiac hypertrophy', *Cell*, 153 (4), 2013, 828–39

Lømo, T., 'The discovery of long-term potentiation', *Philosophical Transactions of the Royal Society of London B*, 358 (1432), 2003, 617–20

Lucey, B. P., and Holtzman, D. M., 'How amyloid, sleep and memory connect', *Nature Neuroscience*, 18 (7), 2015, 933–4

McCay, C. M., Pope, F., Lunsford, W., Sperling, G., Sambhavaphol, P., 'Parabiosis between old and young rats', *Gerontologia*, 1 (1), 1957, 7–17

McEwen, B. S., and Gianaros, P. J., 'Central role of the brain in stress and adaptation: links to socioeconomic status, health, and disease', *Annals of* the *New York Academy of Sciences*, 1186, 2010, 190–222

——, 'Stress- and allostasis-induced brain plasticity', *Annual Review of Medicine*, 62, 2011, 431–45

McGeer, P. L., Itagaki, S., Tago, H., McGeer, E. G., 'Reactive microglia in patients with senile dementia of the Alzheimer type are positive for the histocompatibility glycoprotein HLA-DR', *Neuroscience Letters*, 79 (1–2), 1987, 195–200

Magnusson, S., *Where Memories Go: Why Dementia Changes Everything*, Two Roads, 2015

Mander, B. A., Marks, S. M., Vogel, J. W., Rao, V., Lu, B., Saletin, J. M., . . . Walker, M. P., 'β-amyloid disrupts human NREM slow waves and related hippocampus-dependent memory consolidation', *Nature Neuroscience*, 18 (7), 2015, 1051–7

Mapstone, M., Cheema, A. K., Fiandaca, M. S., Zhong, X., Mhyre, T. R., MacArthur, L. H., . . . Federoff, H. J., 'Plasma phospholipids identify antecedent memory impairment in older adults', *Nature Medicine*, 20 (4), 2014, 415–18

Marcello, E., Gardoni, F., Di Luca, M., 'Alzheimer's disease and modern lifestyle: what is the role of stress?', *Journal of Neurochemistry*, 134 (5), 2015, 795–8

Márquez, G. G., *One Hundred Years of Solitude*, Harper Perennial, 1967

Maurer, K., and Maurer, U., *Alzheimer: The Life of a Physician and the Career of a Disease*, Columbia University Press, 2003

Medawar, P., *Advice to a Young Scientist*, Basic Books, 1981

——, *The Limits of Science*, Oxford University Press, 1985

Merton, R. K., *Science, Technology and Society in Seventeenth-Century England*, Howard Fertig, 2002

Meyer-Luehmann, M., Coomaraswamy, J., Bolmont, T., Kaeser, S., Schaefer, C., Kilger, E., . . . Jucker, M., 'Exogenous induction of cerebral beta-amyloidogenesis is governed by agent and host', *Science*, 313 (5794), 2006, 1781–4

Miklossy, J., 'Alzheimer's disease – a neurospirochetosis. Analysis of the evidence following Koch's and Hill's criteria', *Journal of Neuroinflammation*, 8, 2011, 90

Moran, M., Lynch, C. A., Walsh, C., Coen, R., Coakley, D., Lawlor, B. A., 'Sleep disturbance in mild to moderate Alzheimer's disease', *Sleep Medicine*, 6 (4), 2005, 347–52

Morris, L. G., Veeriah, S., Chan, T. A., 'Genetic determinants at the interface of cancer and neurodegenerative disease', *Oncogene*, 29 (24), 2010, 3453–64

Morris, M., Maeda, S., Vossel, K., Mucke, L., 'The many faces of tau', *Neuron*, 70 (3), 2011, 410–26

Morris, M. C., Tangney, C. C., Wang, Y., Sacks, F. M., Bennett, D. A., Aggarwal, N. T., 'MIND diet associated with reduced incidence of Alzheimer's disease', *Alzheimer's & Dementia*, 11 (9), 2015, 1007–14

Mortimer, J. A., Borenstein, A. R., Gosche, K. M., Snowdon, D. A., 'Very early detection of Alzheimer neuropathology and the role of brain reserve in modifying its clinical expression', *Journal of Geriatric Psychiatry and Neurology*, 18 (4), 2005, 218–22

Motter, R., Vigo-Pelfrey, C., Kholodenko, D., Barbour, R., Johnson-Wood, K., Galasko, D., . . . Schenk, D., 'Reduction of beta-amyloid peptide 42 in the cerebrospinal fluid of patients with Alzheimer's disease', *Annals of Neurology*, 38 (4), 1995, 643–8

Mozolic, J. L., Hayasaka, S., Laurienti, P. J., 'A cognitive training intervention increases resting cerebral blood flow in healthy older adults', *Frontiers in Human Neuroscience*, 4, 2010, 16

Mukherjee, S., *The Emperor of All Maladies: A Biography of Cancer*, Fourth Estate, 2011

——, *Laws of Medicine (TED)*, Simon & Schuster, 2015

——, *The Gene: An Intimate History*, Bodley Head, 2016

Musiek, E. S., and Holtzman, D. M., 'Three dimensions of the amyloid hypothesis: time, space and "wingmen"', *Nature Neuroscience*, 18 (6), 2015, 800–6

Nedergaard, M., 'Garbage truck of the brain', *Science*, 340 (6140), 2013, 1529–30

Nelson, L., Gard, P., Tabet, N., 'Hypertension and inflammation in Alzheimer's disease: close partners in disease development and progression', *Journal of Alzheimer's Disease*, 41 (2), 2014, 331–43

Nelson, L., and Tabet, N., 'Slowing the progression of Alzheimer's disease: what works?', *Ageing Research Reviews*, 23, Pt B, 2015, 193–209

Neri, G., and Opitz, J. M., 'Down syndrome: comments and reflections on the 50th anniversary of Lejeune's discovery', *American Journal of Medical Genetics A*, 149A (12), 2009, 2647–54

Newton, R. D., 'The identity of Alzheimer's disease and senile dementia and their relationship to senility', *British Journal of Psychiatry*, 94 (395), 1948, 225–49

Ngandu, T., Lehtisalo, J., Solomon, A., Levälahti, E., Ahtiluoto, S., Antikainen,

R., . . . Kivipelto, M., 'A 2 year multidomain intervention of diet, exercise, cognitive training, and vascular risk monitoring versus control to prevent cognitive decline in at-risk elderly people (FINGER): a randomised controlled trial', *Lancet*, 385 (9984), 2015, 2255–63

Nicoll, J. A., Wilkinson, D., Holmes, C., Steart, P., Markham, H., Weller, R. O., 'Neuropathology of human Alzheimer disease after immunization with amyloid-beta peptide: a case report', *Nature Medicine*, 9 (4), 448–52

Nimmerjahn, A., Kirchhoff, F., Helmchen, F., 'Resting microglial cells are highly dynamic surveillants of brain parenchyma in vivo', *Science*, 308 (5726), 2005, 1314–18

Noble, D., *The Music of Life: Biology Beyond Genes*, Oxford University Press, 2008

Nordberg, A., Rinne, J. O., Kadir, A., Långström, B., 'The use of PET in Alzheimer disease', *Nature Reviews Neurology*, 6 (2), 2010, 78–87

Office for National Statistics, *Statistical Bulletin: Deaths Registered in England and Wales (Series DR): 2015*, 14 November 2016

Ono, K., Hasegawa, K., Naiki, H., Yamada, M., 'Curcumin has potent anti-amyloidogenic effects for Alzheimer's beta-amyloid fibrils in vitro', *Journal of Neuroscience Research*, 75 (6), 2004, 742–50

Pandav, R., Dodge, H. H., DeKosky, S. T., Ganguli, M., 'Blood pressure and cognitive impairment in India and the United States: a cross-national epidemiological study', *Archives of Neurology*, 60 (8), 2003, 1123–8

Pandav, R., Fillenbaum, G., Ratcliff, G., Dodge, H., Ganguli, M., 'Sensitivity and specificity of cognitive and functional screening instruments for dementia: the Indo-US Cross-National Dementia Epidemiology Study', *Journal of the America Geriatric Society*, 50 (3), 2002, 554–61

Pandav, R., Mehta, A., Belle, S. H., Martin, D. E., Chandra, V., Dodge, H. H., Ganguli, M., 'Data management and quality assurance for an international project: the Indo-US Cross-National Dementia Epidemiology Study', *International Journal of Geriatric Psychiatry*, 17 (6), 2002, 510–18

Park, H. W., 'Longevity, aging, and caloric restriction: Clive Maine McCay and the construction of a multidisciplinary research program', *Historical Studies in the Natural Sciences*, 40 (1), 2010, 79–124

Paul, S. M., and Reddy, K., 'Young blood rejuvenates old brains', *Nature Medicine*, 20 (6), 2014, 582–3

Perlmutter, D., *Grain Brain: The Surprising Truth about Wheat, Carbs, and Sugar – Your Brain's Silent Killers*, Yellow Kite, 2014

Perry, E. K., Perry, R. H., Blessed, G., Tomlinson, B. E., 'Necropsy evidence of central cholinergic deficits in senile dementia', *Lancet*, 1 (8004), 1977, 189

Perry, G., Avila, J., Kinoshita, J., Smith, M. A., *Alzheimer's Disease: A Century of Scientific and Clinical Research*, IOS Press, 2006

Perry, V. H., Nicoll, J. A., Holmes, C., 'Microglia in neurodegenerative disease', *Nature Reviews Neurology*, 6 (4), 2010, 193–201

Pierrot, N., Lhommel, R., Quenon, L., Hanseeuw, B., Dricot, L., Sindic, C., . . . Ivanoiu, A., 'Targretin improves cognitive and biological markers in a patient with Alzheimer's disease, *Journal of Alzheimer's Disease*, 49 (2), 2016, 271–6

Popham, P., 'Dementia: I have a 50:50 chance. But I try not to worry', *Independent*, 16 August 2012

Popovich, P. G., and Longbrake, E. E., 'Can the immune system be harnessed to repair the CNS?', *Nature Reviews Neuroscience*, 9 (6), 2008, 481–93

Popper, K., *The Logic of Scientific Discovery*, Routledge, 2002

Porter, R., *Madness: A Brief History*, Oxford University Press, 2002

Power, R. A., Steinberg, S., Bjornsdottir, G., Rietveld, C. A., Abdellaoui, A., Nivard, M. M., . . . Stefansson, K., 'Polygenic risk scores for schizophrenia and bipolar disorder predict creativity', *Nature Neuroscience*, 18 (7), 2015, 953–5

Pratchett, T., *Shaking Hands with Death*, Penguin, 2014

Prince, M., 'The need for research on dementia in developing countries', *Tropical Medicine & International Health*, 2 (10), 1997, 993–1000

Prince, M., Bryce, R., Ferri, C., 'The benefits of early diagnosis and intervention', Alzheimer's Disease International (ADI), 2011

Prince, M., Comas-Herrera, A., Knapp, M., Guerchet, M., Karagiannidou, M., 'World Alzheimer's Report 2016: Improving healthcare for people living with dementia: coverage, quality and costs now and in the future', Alzheimer's Disease International (ADI), 2016

Prince, M., Wimo, A., Maëlenn, G., Ali G., Wu, Y., Prina, M., 'World Alzheimer Report 2015: The global impact of dementia: an analysis of prevalence, incidence, cost and trends', Alzheimer's Disease International (ADI), 2015

Prusiner, S. B., *Madness and Memory: The Discovery of Prions – A New Biological Principle of Disease*, Yale University Press, 2016

Psaltopoulou T., and Sergentanis, T., 'Mediterranean diet may reduce Alzheimer's risk', *Evidence-based Medicine*, 20 (6), 2015, 202

Raine, C. S., 'Correspondence: re: Robert Terry and Robert Katzman', *Alzheimer's & Dementia*, 1, 2005, 90–1

Ransohoff, R. M., 'Ageing: blood ties', *Nature*, 447, 2011, 41–2

Ratcliff, G., Ganguli, M., Chandra, V., Sharma, S., Belle, S., Seaberg, E., Pandav, R., 'Effects of literacy and education on measures of word fluency', *Brain and Language*, 61 (1), 1998, 115–22

Reagan, R., Proclamation 5565 – National Alzheimer's Disease Month [Filed with the Office of the Federal Register, 11:19 a.m., November 6, 1986], 1986

——, Handwritten letter courtesy of the Ronald Reagan Presidential Foundation and Library, 5 November 1994

Rennie, J., 'The mice that missed: two models for Alzheimer's disease are retracted', *Scientific American*, 1 June 1992

Ridley, M., *Genome: The Autobiography of a Species in 23 Chapters*, Fourth Estate, 2000

Ridley, R. M., Baker, H. F., Windle, C. P., Cummings, R. M., 'Very long term studies of the seeding of beta-amyloidosis in primates', *Journal of Neural Transmission (Vienna)*, 113 (9), 2006, 1243–51

Robakis, N. K., Ramakrishna, N., Wolfe, G., Wisniewski, H. M., 'Molecular cloning and characterization of a cDNA encoding the cerebrovascular and the neuritic plaque amyloid peptides', *Proceedings of the National Academy of Sciences of the United States of America*, 84 (12), 1987, 4190–4

Rockwood, K., Lindsay, J., McDowell, I., 'High blood pressure and dementia', *Lancet*, 348 (9019), 1996, 65–6

Rogaev, E. I., Sherrington, R., Rogaeva, E. A., Levesque, G., Ikeda, M., Liang, Y., . . . St George-Hyslop, P. H., 'Familial Alzheimer's disease in kindreds with missense mutations in a gene on chromosome 1 related to the Alzheimer's disease type 3 gene', *Nature*, 376 (6543), 1995, 775–8

Roh, J. H., Huang, Y., Bero, A. W., Kasten, T., Stewart, F. R., Bateman, R. J., Holtzman, D. M., 'Disruption of the sleep–wake cycle and diurnal fluctuation of β-amyloid in mice with Alzheimer's disease pathology', *Science Translational Medicine*, 4 (150), 2012, 150ra122

Rosca, E. C., Rosca, O., Simu, M., Chirileanu, R. D., 'HIV-associated neuro-cognitive disorders: a historical review', *Neurologist*, 18 (2), 2012, 64–7

Rosén, C., Hansson, O., Blennow, K., Zetterberg, H., 'Fluid biomarkers in Alzheimer's disease – current concepts', *Molecular Neurodegeneration*, 8 (20), 2013, 1–11

Roses, A. D., 'On the discovery of the genetic association of Apolipoprotein E genotypes and common late-onset Alzheimer disease', *Journal of Alzheimer's Disease*, 9, 3 Suppl, 2006, 361–6

Roth, M., Tomlinson, B. E., Blessed, G., 'Correlation between scores for dementia and counts of "senile plaques" in cerebral grey matter of elderly subjects', *Nature*, 209 (5018), 1996, 109–10

Sacks, O., *The Man Who Mistook His Wife for a Hat*, Picador, 2011

——, *The Mind's Eye*, Picador, 2011

——, *Awakenings*, Picador, 2012

St George-Hyslop, P., Haines, J., Rogaev, E., Mortilla, M., Vaula, G., Pericak-Vance, M., . . . Crapper McLachlan, D., 'Genetic evidence for a novel familial Alzheimer's disease locus on chromosome 14', *Nature Genetics*, 2 (4), 1992, 330–4

St George-Hyslop, P. H., Tanzi, R. E., Polinsky, R. J., Haines, J. L., Nee, L., Watkins, P. C., . . . Gusella, J. F., 'The genetic defect causing familial Alzheimer's disease maps on chromosome 21', *Science*, 235 (4791), 1987, 885–90

Sapolsky, R. M., *Why Zebras Don't Get Ulcers*, St Martin's Press, 2004

Saunders, A. M., Strittmatter, W. J., Schmechel, D., George-Hyslop, P. H., Pericak-Vance, M. A., Joo, S. H., . . . Roses, A. D., 'Association of apolipoprotein E allele epsilon 4 with late-onset familial and sporadic Alzheimer's disease', *Neurology*, 43 (8), 1993, 1467–72

Schellenberg, G. D., Bird, T. D., Wijsman, E. M., Orr, H. T., Anderson, L., Nemens, E., . . . Martin, G. M., 'Genetic linkage evidence for a familial Alzheimer's disease locus on chromosome 14', *Science*, 258 (5082), 1992, 668–71

Schenk, D., 'Amyloid-β immunotherapy for Alzheimer's disease: the end of the beginning', *Nature Reviews Neuroscience*, 3, 2002, 824–8

Scudellari, M., 'How iPS cells changed the world', *Nature*, 534 (7607), 2016, 310–12

Selkoe, D. J., Mandelkow, E., Holtzman, D. M, *The Biology of Alzheimer Disease*, Cold Spring Harbor Perspectives in Medicine, 2012

Selye, H., *The Stress of Life*, McGraw-Hill/Schaum's Outlines, 1978

Seok, J., Warren, H. S., Cuenca, A. G., Mindrinos, M. N., Baker, H. V., Xu, W., . . . Host Response to Injury, L. S. C. R. P., 'Genomic responses in mouse models poorly mimic human inflammatory diseases', *Proceedings of the National Academy of Sciences of the United States of America*, 110 (9), 2013, 3507–12

Sepulveda-Falla, D., Glatzel, M., Lopera, F., 'Phenotypic profile of early-onset familial Alzheimer's disease caused by presenilin-1 E280A mutation', *Journal of Alzheimer's Disease*, 32 (1), 2012, 1–12

Shahim, P., Tegner, Y., Wilson, D. H., Randall, J., Skillback, T., Pazooki, D., ... Zetterberg, H., 'Blood biomarkers for brain injury in concussed professional ice hockey players', *JAMA Neurology*, 71 (6), 2014, 684–92

Shelley, M., *Frankenstein: Or, the Modern Prometheus*, Penguin Classics, 2003

Shen, H., 'Studies cast doubt on cancer drug as Alzheimer's treatment', *Nature*, 23 May 2013, online: www.nature.com/news/studies-cast-doubt-on-cancer-drug-as-alzheimer-s-treatment-1.13058

Shenk, D., *The Forgetting: Alzheimer's: Portrait of an Epidemic*, Anchor Books, 2001

Sherrington, R., Rogaev, E. I., Liang, Y., Rogaeva, E. A., Levesque, G., Ikeda, M., ... St George-Hyslop, P. H., 'Cloning of a gene bearing missense mutations in early-onset familial Alzheimer's disease', *Nature*, 375 (6534), 1995, 754–60

Siman, R., Shahim, P., Tegner, Y., Blennow, K., Zetterberg, H., Smith, D. H., 'Serum SNTF increases in concussed professional ice hockey players and relates to the severity of postconcussion symptoms', *Journal of Neurotrauma*, 32 (17), 2015, 1294–300

Singh, B., Parsaik, A. K., Mielke, M. M., Erwin, P. J., Knopman, D. S., Petersen, R. C., Roberts, R. O., 'Association of Mediterranean diet with mild cognitive impairment and Alzheimer's disease: a systematic review and meta-analysis', *Journal of Alzheimer's Disease*, 39 (2), 2014, 271–82

Sinha, M., Jang, Y. C., Oh, J., Khong, D., Wu, E. Y., Manohar, R., ... Wagers, A. J., 'Restoring systemic GDF11 levels reverses age-related dysfunction in mouse skeletal muscle', *Science*, 344 (6184), 2014, 649–52

Small, G. W., Ercoli, L. M., Silverman, D. H., Huang, S. C., Komo, S., Bookheimer, S. Y., ... Phelps, M. E., 'Cerebral metabolic and cognitive decline in persons at genetic risk for Alzheimer's disease', *Proceedings of the National Academy of Sciences of the United States of America*, 97 (11), 2000, 6037–42

Smiley, J., *The Sagas of the Icelanders*, Penguin, 2005

Snowdon, D., *Aging with Grace: The Nun Study and the Science of Old Age. How We Can All Live Longer, Healthier and More Vital Lives*, Fourth Estate, 2011

Soldner, F., and Jaenisch, R., 'iPSC disease modeling', *Science*, 338 (6111), 2012, 1155–6

Solfrizzi, V., Panza, F., Frisardi, V., Seripa, D., Logroscino, G., Imbimbo, B. P., Pilotto, A., 'Diet and Alzheimer's disease risk factors or prevention:

the current evidence', *Expert Reviews of Neurotherapeutics*, 11 (5), 2011, 677–708

Sontag, S., *Illness as Metaphor*, Penguin, 1991

Spinney, L., 'The forgetting gene', *Nature*, 510 (7503), 2014, 26–8

Stadtfeld, M., and Hochedlinger, K., 'Induced pluripotency: history, mechanisms, and applications', *Genes & Development*, 24 (20), 2010, 2239–63

Stamps, J. J., Bartoshuk, L. M., Heilman, K. M., 'A brief olfactory test for Alzheimer's disease', *Journal of the Neurological Sciences*, 333 (1–2), 2013, 19–24

Staropoli, J. F., 'Tumorigenesis and neurodegeneration: two sides of the same coin?', *Bioessays*, 30 (8), 2008, 719–27

Stein, G., *Four in America*, Yale University Press, 1947

Steinberg, M., Leoutsakos, J. M., Podewils, L. J., Lyketsos, C. G., 'Evaluation of a home-based exercise program in the treatment of Alzheimer's disease: the Maximizing Independence in Dementia (MIND) study', *International Journal of Geriatric Psychiatry*, 24 (7), 2009, 680–5

Stern, Y., 'What is cognitive reserve? Theory and research application of the reserve concept', *Journal of the International Neuropsychological Society*, 8 (3), 2002, 448–60

Stossel, S., *My Age of Anxiety*, Windmill Books, 2014

Strittmatter, W. J., Saunders, A. M., Schmechel, D., Pericak-Vance, M., Enghild, J., Salvesen, G. S., Roses, A. D., 'Apolipoprotein E: high-avidity binding to β-amyloid and increased frequency of type 4 allele in late-onset familial Alzheimer disease', *Proceedings of the National Academy of Sciences of the United States of America*, 90 (5), 1993, 1977–81

Summers, W. K., Majovski, L. V., Marsh, G. M., Tachiki, K. Kling, A., 'Oral tetrahydroaminoacridine in long-term treatment of senile dementia, Alzheimer's type', *New England Journal of Medicine*, 315 (20), 1986, 1241–5

Summers, W. K., Viesselman, J. O., Marsh, G. M., Candelora, K., 'Use of THA in treatment of Alzheimer's-like dementia: pilot study in twelve patients', *Biological Psychiatry*, 16 (2), 1981, 145–53

Swaab, D., *We Are Our Brains: From the Womb to Alzheimer's*, Penguin, 2015

Takahashi, K., Tanabe, K., Ohnuki, M., Narita, M., Ichisaka, T., Tomoda, K., Yamanaka, S., 'Induction of pluripotent stem cells from adult human fibroblasts by defined factors', *Cell*, 131 (5), 2007, 861–72

Takahashi, K., and Yamanaka, S., 'Induction of pluripotent stem cells from mouse embryonic and adult fibroblast cultures by defined factors', *Cell*, 126 (4), 2006, 663–76

Tang, H., Hammack, C., Ogden, S. C., Wen, Z., Qian, X., Li, Y., . . . Ming, G. L., 'Zika virus infects human cortical neural progenitors and attenuates their growth', *Cell Stem Cell*, 18 (5), 2016, 587–90

Tanzi, R. E., *Decoding Darkness: The Search for the Genetic Causes of Alzheimer's Disease*, Perseus, 2001

——, 'A brief history of Alzheimer's disease gene discovery', *Journal of Alzheimer's Disease*, 33 Suppl 1, 2013, S5–13

Tanzi, R. E., and Bertram, L., 'Twenty years of the Alzheimer's disease amyloid hypothesis: a genetic perspective', *Cell*, 120 (4), 545–55

Tanzi, R. E., Gusella, J., Watkins, P. C., Bruns, G. A., St George-Hyslop, P., Van Keuren, M. L., . . . Neve, R. L., 'Amyloid beta protein gene: cDNA, mRNA distribution, and genetic linkage near the Alzheimer locus', *Science*, 235 (4791), 1987, 880–4

Taylor, B., *The Last Asylum: A Memoir of Madness in Our Times*, Penguin, 2015

Taylor, M., Moore, S., Mourtas, S., Niarakis, A., Re, F., Zona, C., . . . Allsop, D., 'Effect of curcumin-associated and lipid ligand-functionalized nanoliposomes on aggregation of the Alzheimer's Aβ peptide', *Nanomedicine: Nanotechnology, Biology, and Medicine*, 7 (5), 2011, 541–50

Terry, R. D., Gonatas, N. K., Weiss, M., 'Ultrastructural studies in Alzheimer's presenile dementia', *American Journal of Pathology*, 44, 1964, 269–97

Thelma, B. K., Juyal, R. C., Dodge, H. H., Pandav, R., Chandra, V., Ganguli, M., 'APOE polymorphism in a rural older population-based sample in India', *Human Biology*, 73 (1), 2001, 135–44

Thomson, J. A., Itskovitz-Eldor, J., Shapiro, S. S., Waknitz, M. A., Swiergiel, J. J., Marshall, V. S., Jones, J. M., 'Embryonic stem cell lines derived from human blastocysts', *Science*, 282 (5391), 1998, 1145–7

UK Department of Health, 'Dementia: A State of the Nation Report on Dementia Care and Support in England', 29 November 2013

Underwood, E., 'Alzheimer's amyloid theory gets modest boost', *Science*, 349 (6247), 2015, 464

Van Broeckhoven, C., Backhovens, H., Cruts, M., De Winter, G., Bruyland, M., Cras, P., Martin, J. J., 'Mapping of a gene predisposing to early-onset Alzheimer's disease to chromosome 14q24.3', *Nature Genetics*, 2 (4), 1992, 335–9

Van de Winckel, A., Feys, H., De Weerdt, W., Dom, R., 'Cognitive and behavioural effects of music-based exercises in patients with dementia', *Clinical Rehabilitation*, 18 (3), 2004, 253–60

Van der Worp, H. B., Howells, D. W., Sena, E. S., Porritt, M. J., Rewell, S., O'Collins, V., Macleod, M. R., 'Can animal models of disease reliably inform human studies?', *PLoS Medicine*, 7 (3), 2010, e1000245

Vassar, R., 'BACE1 inhibitor drugs in clinical trials for Alzheimer's disease', *Alzheimer's Research and Therapy*, 6 (9), 2014, 89

Verghese, A., *The New York Times Book of Medicine: More Than 150 Years of Reporting on the Evolution of Medicine*, Sterling, 2015

Verkhratsky, A., and Butt, A., *Glial Neurobiology*, John Wiley, 2007

Villeda, S. A., Luo, J., Mosher, K. I., Zou, B., Britschgi, M., Bieri, G., . . . Wyss-Coray, T., 'The ageing systemic milieu negatively regulates neurogenesis and cognitive function', *Nature*, 477 (7362), 2011, 90–4

Villeda, S. A., Plambeck, K. E., Middeldorp, J., Castellano, J. M., Mosher, K. I., Luo, J., . . . Wyss-Coray, T., 'Young blood reverses age-related impairments in cognitive function and synaptic plasticity in mice', *Nature Medicine*, 20 (6), 2014, 659–63

Von Radowitz, J., 'Vampire therapy: young blood may reverse ageing', *Independent*, 4 May 2014

Vonnegut, K., *Cat's Cradle*, Penguin Classics, 2008

Wade, N., 'Thomas S. Kuhn: Revolutionary Theorist of Science', *Science*, 197 (4299), 1977, 143–5

Wang, S. S., 'Alzheimer's families clamor for drug', *Wall Street Journal*, 11 February 2012

Warren, H. S., Tompkins, R. G., Moldawer, L. L., Seok, J., Xu, W., Mindrinos, M. N., . . . Davis, R. W., 'Mice are not men', *Proceedings of the National Academy of Sciences of the United States of America*, 112 (4), 2015, E345

Watkins, C. C., and Treisman, G. J., 'Cognitive impairment in patients with AIDS – prevalence and severity', *HIV AIDS*, 7, 2015, 35–47

Watson, J., *The Double Helix*, Weidenfeld & Nicolson, 2011

Weingarten, M. D., Lockwood, A. H., Hwo, S. Y., Kirschner, M. W., 'A protein factor essential for microtubule assembly', *Proceedings of the National Academy of Sciences*, 72 (5), 1975, 1858–62

Weissman, I. L., 'The road ended up at stem cells', *Immunological Reviews*, 185, 2002, 159–74

White, L., Petrovitch, H., Ross, G. W., Masaki, K. H., Abbott, R. D., Teng, E. L., . . . Curb, J. D., 'Prevalence of dementia in older Japanese-American men in Hawaii: the Honolulu-Asia Aging Study', *Journal of American Medical Association*, 276 (12), 1996, 955–60

Whitlock, J. R., Sutherland, R. J., Witter, M. P., Moser, M. B., Moser, E. I.,

'Navigating from hippocampus to parietal cortex', *Proceedings of the National Academy of Sciences of the United States of America*, 105 (39), 2009, 14755–62

Wilson, R. S., Arnold, S. E., Schneider, J. A., Kelly, J. F., Tang, Y., Bennett, D. A., 'Chronic psychological distress and risk of Alzheimer's disease in old age', *Neuroepidemiology*, 27 (3), 2006, 143–53

Wilson, R. S., Barnes, L., Bennett, D. A., Li, Y., Bienias, J. L., Mendes de Leon, C. F., Evans, D. A., 'Proneness to psychological distress and risk of Alzheimer disease in a biracial community', *Neurology*, 64 (2), 2005, 380–2

Wilson, R. S., Evans, D. A., Bienias, J. L., Mendes de Leon, C. F., Schneider, J. A., Bennett, D. A., 'Proneness to psychological distress is associated with risk of Alzheimer's disease', *Neurology*, 61 (11), 2003, 1479–85

Wilson, R. S., Mendes de Leon, C. F., Barnes, L. L., Schneider, J. A., Bienias, J. L., Evans, D. A., Bennett, D. A., 'Participation in cognitively stimulating activities and risk of incident Alzheimer disease', *Journal of the American Medical Association*, 287 (6), 2002, 742–8

Winblad, B., and Blum, K. I., 'Hints of a therapeutic vaccine for Alzheimer's?', *Neuron*, 38 (4), 2003, 517–18

Wise, J., 'Blood test can predict Alzheimer's disease, say US scientists', *British Medical Journal*, 348, 2014, g2074

Wiseman, F. K., Al-Janabi, T., Hardy, J., Karmiloff-Smith, A., Nizetic, D., Tybulewicz, V. L., . . . Strydom, A., 'A genetic cause of Alzheimer disease: mechanistic insights from Down syndrome', *Nature Reviews Neuroscience*, 16 (9), 2015, 564–74

Wolpert, L., *Malignant Sadness: The Anatomy of Depression*, Free Press, 2000
——, *How We Live and Why We Die: The Secret Lives of Cells*, Faber & Faber, 2010

Wood, H., 'Alzheimer disease: evidence for trans-synaptic and exo-synaptic tau propagation in Alzheimer disease', *Nature Reviews Neurology*, 11 (12), 2015, 665

World Health Organization (WHO), 'Dementia: Fact Sheet', April 2016

Wright, D. E., Wagers, A. J., Gulati, A. P., Johnson, F. L., Weissman, I. L., 'Physiological migration of hematopoietic stem and progenitor cells', *Science*, 294 (5548), 2001, 1933–6

Yaffe, K. D., Vittinghoff, E., Lindquist, K., Barnes, D., Covinsky, K., Neylan, T., . . . Marmar, C., 'Post-traumatic stress disorder and risk of dementia among U.S. veterans', *Archives of General Psychiatry*, 67 (6), 2010, 608–13

Yaguez, L., Shaw, K. N., Morris, R., Matthews, D., 'The effects on cognitive functions of a movement-based intervention in patients with Alzheimer's type dementia: a pilot study', *International Journal of Geriatric Psychiatry*, 26 (2), 2011, 173–81

Yang, F., Lim, G. P., Begum, A. N., Ubeda, O. J., Simmons, M. R., Ambegaokar, S. S., . . . Cole, G. M., 'Curcumin inhibits formation of amyloid beta oligomers and fibrils, binds plaques, and reduces amyloid in vivo', *Journal of Biological Chemistry*, 280 (7), 2005, 5892–901

Yang, J., Li, S., He, X. B., Cheng, C., Le, W., 'Induced pluripotent stem cells in Alzheimer's disease: applications for disease modeling and cell-replacement therapy', *Molecular Neurodegeneration*, 11 (1), 2016, 39

Zetterberg, H., and Blennow, K., 'Cerebrospinal fluid biomarkers for Alzheimer's disease: more to come?', *Journal of Alzheimer's Disease*, 33 Suppl 1, 2013, S361–9

Zissimopoulos, J., Crimmins, E., St Clair, P., 'The value of delaying Alzheimer's disease onset', *Forum for Health Economics and Policy*, 18 (1), 2014, 25–39

Zlokovic, B. V., 'The blood-brain barrier in health and chronic neuro-degenerative disorders', *Neuron*, 57 (2), 2008, 178–201

Index

AD in subentries refers to Alzheimer's disease

From Byron, Austen and Darwin

to some of the most acclaimed and original
contemporary writing, John Murray takes pride in
bringing you powerful, prizewinning, absorbing
and provocative books that will entertain you
today and become the classics of tomorrow.

We put a lot of time and passion into what we
publish and how we publish it, and we'd like to
hear what you think.

Be part of John Murray – share your views with us at:

www.johnmurray.co.uk
 johnmurraybooks
@johnmurrays
johnmurraybooks